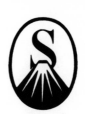

OTHER BOOKS BY
BEN E. BENJAMIN, Ph.D.

*Are You Tense?*

# SPORTS WITHOUT PAIN

## BEN E. BENJAMIN, Ph.D.

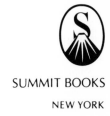

SUMMIT BOOKS

NEW YORK

Copyright © 1979 by Ben E. Benjamin, Ph.D.
All rights reserved
including the right of reproduction
in whole or in part in any form
Published by *Summit Books*
A Simon & Schuster Division of Gulf & Western Corporation
Simon & Schuster Building
1230 Avenue of the Americas
New York, New York 10020

*Designed by Stanley S. Drate*
Manufactured in the United States of America

1 2 3 4 5 6 7 8 9 10


Library of Congress Cataloging in Publication Data

Benjamin, Ben E., Ph.D. date.
    Sports without pain.

    1. Physical fitness. 2. Exercise. 3. Sports—Physiological aspects. I. Title.
GV481.B46      613.7'1      78-11188

ISBN: 0-671-40064-9

To Dr. Barbara G. Koopman
In gratitude for her help
and encouragement
in my movement toward life

# ACKNOWLEDGMENTS

It's difficult to make acknowledgments interesting, because they relate to only a few people. Many people worked hard in helping this book come together. First, I'd like to thank my fellow students at Union Graduate School for encouraging me to do this book. I'd also like to thank Colin Greer for his encouragement and for recommending my agent, Liz Darhansoff. Her steadfast efforts got me the best publisher I could have hoped for. My thanks to Beth Lind for her assistance in solidifying my original ideas, and for helping me write the initial proposal. My appreciation to Jim Silberman, a publisher with foresight, and to Chris Steinmetz, my editor, for her help in expanding and clarifying the focus of this book. No writer could have had a more enthusiastic and reasonable editor.

Thanks to Ara Fitzgerald and Jim Finney for their assistance in writing some of the first draft, and to Joe Aliaga for his writing and technical assistance. My appreciation to Sylvia Bhourne for her endless retyping, and to my secretary, Janna Jensen, for her untiring Xeroxing.

My thanks to Paula Josef for her wonderful drawings and to Harold Zipkowitz for his lovely photographs. My thanks to Colette Blonigan and Mike Welsh, who happily posed for the photographs. My thanks to Drs. Herskowitz, Koopman, Liebler, Weingrad, and Ross for their suggestions upon reviewing the final manuscript. Also, my gratitude to

Bena Kallick, Mary Sheerin, Ann Ladd, and Signe Lundberg for their criticisms and encouragements, and to Lea Delacour for her precise critiques and moral support. I'd also like to thank all of my students for contributing to my education.

My thanks to the following people for their help and advice:

Michael Altabet; Bob Barrow; Don Berk; Steve Ruma; David Bryant; Norman Campbell; Gregory Castro; Steve Cochran; Robert Cook, M.D.; Jerry Cooke; Vern Cordier; Mike Dawkins; Art Diemar; Molly Fleming; Sandy Goodman; Jerry Hauck; Dale Helley; Gregory Jones; Gretchen Langstaff; Eliza Mallouk; Gary Millennor; Pamela Matti; Gary Nelson; Dale Pritchard; Troy Reynolds; Ray Rippman; Linda Roberts; Carmen Salvino; Felix Samarron; Chuck Stanley; Peter Stephan; Mary Vait; Danny Whelan; Joanne Widness; Nancy Wold.

My thanks to Carol Hess for her love, encouragement, and continual assistance in rewriting and rewriting. My gratitude to Perry White for his endless efforts in helping write draft after draft, for his continuous and honest criticism, and for his ability to aid, rather than inhibit, my creative thrust. My deep thanks to Carol Boggs for so many things: for her help in clarifying and rewriting the chapters on alignment and strength; for collaborating with me in creating the stretching, strength-building and alignment exercises; for permitting me the use of the many fine exercises and concepts that she has developed; and for the fun we had in working together. Finally, my deep gratitude to Leonard J. Smith for his relentless efforts in forcing me to clarify, reconsider, and rewrite nearly everything of importance. I'd also like to thank him for his guidance in the development of my entire career.

# CONTENTS

# EXERCISES

## II. TENSION-RELAXATION EXERCISES

## IV. STRENGTH-BUILDING EXERCISES

## V.  ALIGNMENT EXERCISES

# SPORTS WITHOUT PAIN

# 1

# WHAT DO YOU HAVE
# TO FEAR?

Relax! You may be among the 10 percent of professional and amateur athletes who exercise and never receive a major injury or even the usual minor pains and discomforts many people get. If you are among the other 90 percent, just listen! The odds are that within the next few years, two out of every three persons involved in a sport or some form of exercise will sustain a major injury or at least several minor ones. Pulled hamstrings, sprained ligaments, painful knees, torn cartilages, spasms of the back and legs, aching joints, and shooting pains are just some of the problems that may plague you. This can happen if you ignore the simple laws governing the use of your body, laws which many of the greatest professional athletes don't even know and understand.

The greatest fear of a professional athlete is that he will incur an injury which could weaken his potential or bring his career to a premature end. It can never be known what heights of accomplishment could have been reached by a Joe Namath or an O. J. Simpson in football, by a Mickey Mantle in baseball, if they hadn't been plagued by ailments which blocked the full expression of their extraordinary talents. What incredible records could have been set by lefty pitcher Sandy Koufax or by Willis Reed in basketball if their careers had not come to a grinding halt due to physical disabilities. Is it strictly a matter of luck, as many spectators believe, that some athletes suffer disabling setbacks while others incur few, if any, serious injuries? There is room for doubt.

But aren't serious injuries more likely to happen to professional athletes in competitive sports rather than to amateurs? The answer is *no!* For example, one out of every twenty skiers has a serious accident every season. Thousands of joggers suffer knee or ankle pain each year, and hundreds of thousands of tennis players will suffer tennis elbow next season. These facts only scratch the surface of the possibilities for painful discomfort and loss of pleasure, time, and money. But isn't the risk of injury, either minor or major, something that one must accept if he chooses to participate in athletic activities? Again, isn't it a matter of luck, chance, or circumstance? Not entirely. Let's take a look at the professional athlete who does manage to escape repeated injury.

For ten years one of the greatest fullbacks of all time, Jim Brown of the Cleveland Browns, went through a full career without suffering one major injury—a remarkable achievement when one considers that the meanest defensive linemen in football zeroed in on Brown when their teams played Cleveland, because to stop him meant almost sure victory. How did Brown escape the odds? There are hints: He was the slowest walker, not runner, to and from a huddle; he was also the slowest riser after being tackled; when running he appeared deceptively fast because his rhythm was sure and his speed appropriate to the circumstances—if the opening was small, he had the needed burst of energy to cut through, and in open field running he possessed a smooth, flowing movement which only increased if a tackle neared. He knew when to use and conserve his energy. The resilient yielding of his body when hit by other bodies was right for the moment.

How did Walt Frazier, the great basketball player of the New York Knicks, avoid a major injury in a full career of fast, exacting competition? Again, one is struck by Frazier's deceptive speed and his wise use of energy. As in Brown's case, there was softness rather than hardness, a sense of what was needed and what was not, and no sign of overexertion or stiff movement, but rather that paradoxical combination of restful action, gentle aggression, and yielding, resilient defense.

Obviously, a physical and mental attitude which helped reduce the prospects of injury was at work for these men. Both of them have a natural ability which helped them avoid serious injury. Most of us are not so endowed, but we can protect ourselves from serious and repeated injury by adequate training and preparation. The time is long overdue to focus on exercises which could benefit the layman and the professional athlete in cutting down unnecessary risks leading to pain and injury.

Throughout this book, I ask you to keep in mind the incredible career accomplishments of people like Jim Brown in football, Walt Frazier in basketball, Rod Laver in tennis, Jean Claude Killy in skiing, and the other 10 percent of all of us who are able to exercise without fear. I am going to show how sports and exercise can be beneficial and pleasurable with a minimum risk of pain and injury, and I will point out which exercises may be good for you, which may not, and why. Let's look at what may happen to you if you don't exercise properly.

Exercise is good for you. This is a fact. Doctors, nutritionists, athletes, secretaries, businessmen, housewives, and even people who don't regularly exercise agree. We all feel the effects of the fact that physical exertion has been virtually eliminated in our modernized society, so more and more people who lead sedentary lives are rediscovering the joys and benefits of activities like jogging, tennis, basketball, skiing, exercise classes, or whatever else strikes their fancy.

Unless you treat your body properly, however, it is very likely that you will encounter that one element which has crept in and ruined many athletic careers—injury. In the excitement and sweat of sports and exercise that we enjoy, we often forget that we are not invincible. It is exciting to discover that our bodies can bend, yet devastating when you learn that they can also break. You could literally be one step away from pain, injury, or a crippling "accident" that can prevent you from ever doing vigorous exercise again.

Injury may mean that you will be crippled for the season or for a year or so, or it may mean that you will never be able to play your favorite sport again. You may be left suffering with severe pain, which certainly takes the pleasure out of exercise. Worst of all, you may have to have surgery. In the United States alone, there are many thousands of back and knee operations every year that might have been avoided. Seven million people receive some kind of treatment for back pain every day of each year, and one out of every three adults is plagued by pain every single day.*

*Finneson, Bernard E., M.D., with Dr. Arthur S. Freese. *The New Approach to Lower Back Pain.* New York: Berkley Publishing Corp., 1975, pp 46–47

Injury has several side effects. If you have a serious injury, you will probably never play quite as well again, and you will be continually frustrated. With every injury, except for a broken bone that has healed properly, you become more vulnerable to reinjuring that area or an adjacent one. Often you must move differently to compensate for the injured area, which can create accumulations of muscle tension and probable reinjury.

There are always new dangers. If you don't exercise a part of your body for a short period of time, the muscles begin to shrink and weaken in a natural process called atrophy. And if you try to come back too fast, as many people do, you may reinjure that same vulnerable knee or elbow, usually causing a worse problem the second time around. You might be left with chronic weaknesses increasing the possibility of strain and further injury.

Injury often leaves its victims with deep fears, so that they constantly hold themselves back from letting go. It creates tensions within you—you get so obsessed with being careful that your movements become restrained. You can't become totally immersed in the activity, ready to spring into action. You may forever hesitate. Your game will slow down. It will be difficult and perhaps impossible to regain that feeling of being lost in the excitement of that basketball game or tennis match.

You don't *have* to get injured if you like to run or play tennis. You can lessen the risks easily if you spend just a little time taking care of yourself. If you prepare your body before sports and exercise, and if you exercise regularly, your body will be more resilient, flexible, and strong, and less vulnerable to pain and injury. The better you take care of yourself, the longer your exercise life will be. Vigorous exercise should be part of your life. It is often dangerous, but it need not be, and that is what this book is about.

The exercises in this book were developed over the past fifteen years through my private practice and workshops I have taught throughout the country. At the Muscular Therapy Institute, I have worked with thousands of people suffering from pain and injury, often as a direct result of postural alignment and tension problems. With my colleagues I have designed numerous exercise programs to help people from all walks of life learn how to overcome these problems and exercise without fear of injury. These exercises have been tested over many years, and are safe and painless.

This book offers a highly effective exercise warm-up program for every sport. If you follow the simple directions, you can improve your performance and protect yourself from getting injured. In addition, there is a fitness profile to help you identify your body's most vulnerable areas. Once you are familiar with these you can select strength-building, stretching, alignment, and tension-release exercises designed to correct your particular problems. Then you can create an individualized warm-up program suited to the needs of your own body by using specific exercises for your problem areas along with the general warm-ups given. For easy reference, the exercises in each chapter are subdivided according to specific parts of the body.

# 2

# MAKING COMMON SENSE COMMON

The most important aspect of preparing for an exercise or sports program is to use your own common sense about what you do. Before we explore the specific warm-up program which will help you play better and avoid injury, here are some simple guidelines that everyone should follow in his or her sports program.

## PLEASURE YOURSELF

That's what it's all about—pleasuring yourself. Doing something that makes you feel good. Participate in an exercise program or a sport that you enjoy. The only exception is when the exercises you like are not good for you, such as running when you have chronic knee pain. Whether your physical activity is for fun, or for your lower-back pain, or cardiovascular reconditioning, it should always be something that you enjoy.

If you don't like doing something, you probably won't be able to do it well. Not only does forced activity create a lot of tension, but it's simply unnecessary. There are lots of ways to get proper exercise. If you like to swim and you hate to run, swim. If you don't like sports but like to dance, dance. If you find exercise programs boring or lonely, then actively try to find a sport that satisfies you. Try experimenting with different ones. If you keep looking and trying, you will find an activity that suits you.

## PAIN IS A FRIENDLY SIGNAL

Pain is one of the most valuable feelings you can ever get. It is part of the language of your body. It tells you when something is wrong, and tells you how wrong it is by the degree of pain you experience. Brief pain can be a warning of worse things to come if you don't listen and respond. Intense or constant pains are loud, clear announcements to stop or else. Or else what? The body often contracts violently and hurts to prevent you from a continued action that might tear a tendon, sprain a ligament, turn a minor bone fracture into a severe break, sever a nerve, or stop your heart. Pain is your lifesaver. When your body talks, listen. Learn to understand the messages that your body gives you. They may be precautionary messages like "Continue but slow down," or "Jack, take a break before you go on," "Mary, warm up some more," or "Harry, you're eighty-five. Give up tennis already." But on the other hand, your body's message might be urgently saying, "Jane, don't move, your leg is fractured," or "Sorry, Jim, you will have to lie in bed for three weeks because of what you did to your lower back with that piano moving."

When you have pain anywhere in your body, don't ignore it. Investigate it. Just use your head—if your pain is slight and goes away with a little rest, that's fine. But if it's severe or constantly recurring, get some help. Whenever you are unsure of what your body pain is saying, call your doctor. The motto I teach is: *If it hurts, don't do it.* It's better to be safe than incapacitated for years, or the rest of your life, because you would not listen. It's your body—no one else cares about it more than you do. Take care of it because it has to last you awhile.

## FOLLOW YOUR FEELINGS

There are three aspects to following your feelings. One is knowing whether to do it or not. Another is knowing when to stop. The third is knowing when to go easy. For example, when you're downhill skiing and the mountain calls you for one last run at 3:30—should you go? That depends on whether you are feeling strong and not fatigued. If you feel tired but go anyway—watch out. The snow may be wetter and your skis will turn with greater difficulty, as many "hot dogs" have found racing down the beginner's slope just as the lift line closes only to complete their last run on a stretcher. Or you may be in the middle of a tennis match and your shoulder begins to hurt. What should you do? Many will try to ignore it in the excitement of competition, but there are two alternatives: Tell your partner what's happened and graciously bow out, or take it easy and concentrate on your tactics rather than your power.

Don't force yourself to exercise when you don't feel like it. Compulsive activity often leads to injury. If you don't really feel like exercising one day, it's a good idea to forget it and try again the next day. If you have a strong resistance to moving that day and you exercise, you will not be as alert, your reaction time will slow down, and the likelihood of getting hurt will increase. Even if you're in the middle of a game, or you've done your warm-up, or you've just gotten to the park and you are ready to jog, listen to yourself, respect yourself, stop and call it a day. Challenge the resistance only if it is small, if you recognize it as an old friend that needs a little push in order to feel great again. It's true that if you didn't exercise every time you felt a little resistant to it you might not ever do anything. There is a part of everyone that would prefer to just sit and vegetate in the security of inactivity. Obviously, this is not good and should be overcome. Inertia is a powerful force.

True, it's often more difficult to stop when you're playing with someone else, but you must learn to know when to quit. Trying to live up to other people's expectations at the expense of your health sets you up for injury. It is your responsibility to follow your feelings. If you don't take care of yourself, no one else will.

## TAKING BREAKS

When you exercise a muscle too long, it uses up its oxygen supply and gets fatigued. If you take breaks, you can go for a longer time at your favorite sport. Just resting for two to four minutes after a half-hour of tennis gives your body a chance to recover enough to make the second half-hour a lot easier. The second way to take a break is to use the opposite set of muscles. For example, alternating swimming on your front and on your back, or volleying with your left hand in between tennis matches, gives your body some needed variation in movement to allow the muscles used in your primary activity to recover. It also helps your muscles to develop more evenly. Don't be compulsive. Give yourself a break. A few minutes of rest will give you fifteen to twenty minutes of more pleasure with greater safety.

## SORENESS

A slight feeling of soreness occasionally is normal. But to always feel sore after exercising is a sure sign that something's wrong. When you begin an activity that your body isn't used to, you may get a little sore the next day. If you get extremely sore, you're doing too much too soon. Slow down.

Soreness occurs when muscle fibers are slightly strained or torn. This can result from extreme overexertion or from activity that's too demanding on the available capillary beds. What's happening is that you are building up new muscle tissue by increasing the demand on your body. To the extent that a muscle has been inactive, the capillaries can't provide enough blood to equal the new demand. When you don't use a muscle, some of the capillaries which carry the blood dry up and disappear. Once you begin to exercise there's a sudden need for more of these small blood vessels to re-form. The problem is that it takes five or six times as long to redevelop the blood supply as it does to develop the muscle. That's why if you wish to avoid painful soreness, you have to build up slowly. A little soreness is okay, but not more than that.

The body sometimes reacts to a new activity by contracting slightly. This also causes an achey or sore feeling. When this occurs you have two choices that can enhance the repair process. You can rest for a few days and renew your activity more gradually, or you can exercise gently, stretching easily or using moderate strength-building exercises.

An important reason why people get sore is simply that they don't warm up. If you don't prepare your body before vigorous activity, you will tend to strain your muscles. Proper warm-up will often eliminate minor soreness from exercising.

Excess tension causes frequent soreness after exercise. Muscles that are tense bear a double load when you exercise them, because you are using only part of your energy to do the work itself and are using the rest of your energy to keep the muscles in a state of unnecessary contraction. This often leads to strain, premature fatigue, and microscopic tears in the muscle. When muscles become sore very easily it is often a sign of chronic fatigue. Exercising with tense and sore muscles is like driving a car with the brakes on. Torn and pulled muscles, spasms, and tendon injuries are common in people who are chronically sore because of tension.

## STITCH PAIN

Clients often say to me, "I frequently get a stitch pain in my side when I run. What does that mean?" A stitch pain in the side results from a spasm of the diaphragm, which is the muscle primarily responsible for breathing. It usually results from demanding too much work from your breathing apparatus without preparation. If you begin to run when you are especially tense, the diaphragm tends to quickly reach its metabolic limit. When this happens it contracts, which is a painful way of telling you to stop. Unless you're very tense, a proper warm-up will usually eliminate stitch pain completely. Stitch pain can occur even though you do the same activity at other times without any problem.

The next question usually is, "Should I run through it, or stop?" Running through a stitch pain is not a good idea. More fibers of the diaphragm muscle can become involved, and doing this might cause you to strain the diaphragm. I suggest that you walk or jog very slowly for four to five minutes to see whether or not the spasm releases. If the pain is gone, then slowly increase your speed. If the stitch pain does return, stop! Your body is telling you that you've had enough. The warm-up program outlined in this book can greatly reduce the likelihood of stitch pain.

## FRESH AIR AND LIGHT

Ours is one of the few civilizations whose citizens spend nine-tenths of their lives indoors and sitting. We're usually outside to and from work, and maybe for a few hours on the weekends. When you exercise, you have a golden opportunity to get outside. Whenever you have a choice, go outdoors. Summer, winter, spring, or fall, your body can use air and light.

It is no accident that in track and field events, records of outdoor meet running times are superior to indoor track records. Besides the natural resiliency of the earth as opposed to the hard, less yielding indoor surfaces, the fact that the air indoors is never as fresh as outdoors does affect performance levels. Within any enclosure you get an accumulation of smoke and heavy air from crowds breathing in a contained environment. This cuts down on oxygen and contributes to a greater strain on the body and thus to slower running times. Baseball players in the National League often refer to the pleasure of playing in the only ball park without lights, Wrigley Field in Chicago. They say quite simply that it feels better to play in daylight than at night; it feels more natural. Any sports fan can verify how much more relaxing and pleasurable it is to watch an afternoon baseball game than a night game, how much more pleasurable it is to observe any outdoor sports event like a soccer match or football game as opposed to going into an enclosed arena. The addition of artificial factors affects all physical activities adversely: from artificial turf in baseball and football, which has increased the number of serious injuries, to the dulling, suppressive effect of artificial light.

Of course, due to weather conditions and the inaccessibility of many forms of exercise paraphernalia in the outdoors, it is necessary to compromise, to use indoor places for some forms of exercise. But outdoor exercise is preferable, and to the extent that it is feasible it should be sought and made a part of one's life.


## NOT EVERYBODY IS AN EXPERT

When we have a tax problem, we see an accountant. When the lights go out, we call an electrician. But when we have a pain in the back we ask the butcher, the plumber, a friend, or anyone we know who's had it.

One client of mine, who was a jogger, came in with severe pain in the front lower leg. His pain had been getting worse consistently for a year. In speaking to his athletic coach he was advised to run longer distances at a slower pace. I sent him to his physician to ask for X-rays before I would treat him. He called me and told me that his X-rays showed nine hairline fractures of the tibia, the lower leg bone.

In another case, a gymnast attended one of my self-care workshops recently and said she had been suffering from a pulled hamstring for about nine months. When I asked her what she had done for it, she told me she had diligently followed her fellow students' advice and tried to stretch out her hamstrings every day. She was surprised to learn that what she was doing perpetuated her injury. By stretching her torn muscle fibers daily she never permitted them to knit and heal. In actuality, she reinjured herself every day.

Often the last person we ask is the doctor. Everybody's problem is different. With identical symptoms of low back pain one could have a back spasm or a tumor on the spine, a sprained ligament or a ruptured disc. In some cases, the loss of time and the lack of restriction of movement or activity could be crucial or even fatal.

If your bones or joints hurt, see an orthopedist or a neurologist. If you don't know whom to see, call your family doctor. If you don't have one, call a major hospital in your area and ask for help.

## KNOW YOUR AGE AND WHAT IT MEANS

Your body grows and develops until you are about twenty-five. This period of your life is considered your youth. Up to that time the body can take almost anything. Around age twenty-five the body slowly begins to break down. That doesn't mean that you can't be in good shape as you get older. I expect to live and to work until I'm at least one hundred years old. What it means is that you have to take better and better care of yourself as you get older if you want to remain active and in good health.

Around age twenty-five, when the mature years begin, your body stops its growth process and subtle physiological changes start to take place. Thousands of brain cells die every day, more of your ligament fibers change from elastic to rigid, and by the time you reach age seventy your bones become less dense and can support only one-fifth of the weight that they could when you were twenty-five.

It's all very natural, so don't fight it—go with it. At fifty you can't do what you did if you were in good shape at twenty-five. If you try to, the possibility of injury is very great. However, if you were in bad shape at twenty-five you might even be able to do more at fifty if you are in good condition.

## SPORTS AND PAINKILLING DRUGS

Sports and drugs are bad news. If you want to avoid injury, listen to your pain and what your body tells you. If you like danger and want to court injury, mix drugs with sports. When you close your eyes and stuff your bills into a drawer and don't pay them, you pay later, and with interest. Don't exercise today and sacrifice your health for the rest of your life. Exercising while taking painkilling drugs is like hiding from the truth. If your body tells you to stop, then stop—it has its reasons. If you inject the muscle, pop a pill, or freeze-spray your spasm, you take the chance of paying a heavy price. We've seen it happen time after time in professional sports when an athlete plays right after a cortisone injection to the knee, shoulder, or elbow, only to end up suffering further injury. Highly paid professionals such as Willis Reed in basketball, Joe Namath in football, Sandy Koufax in baseball, or Billie Jean King in tennis have had this happen to them. Painkillers cannot and do not prevent increased vulnerability to injury.

If it's your profession to get out there on the field or on the stage, and you know that your career can be cut short and filled with injuries and pain, and you accept this, then by all means go ahead. I'm not saying that drugs are inherently evil. Medicine has discovered many fine drugs that stop pain, increase healing, and help us in many important ways. However, the pervasive and inordinate use of drugs that numb us to our bodies' sensations so that we can perform vigorous, stressful tasks makes us incredibly vulnerable to serious injury. You do have a choice.

When you take a drug, not all of your faculties are completely available to you, you're less in touch with your body, and therefore you react slower. Or you will do something that your body's pain and contraction are telling you not to do and you will probably end up ripping or tearing a ligament or tendon. I have seen many athletes' and dancers' careers shattered dramatically by just such an event. Listen to your body. The muscles contract and hurt to tell you to stop before more serious things happen.

The point is that when you feel a pain it's a warning to stop. If you're numbed to these signals by drugs, you won't know when to stop and will go past the signal and get injured.

## PATIENCE

Impatience is surely one of the biggest causes of injury. In exercise, as well as in many other areas of life, change must happen slowly if it is to be deep and lasting. You want your body to change fast but it resists abrupt change, it doesn't like it. If you demand new things from your body too quickly, it will rebel.

When you decide to take up exercising or to learn a new sport, you often start with a "gung-ho" attitude, but enthusiasm soon peters out. The reason: "It wasn't exciting enough," or "I wasn't good at it," or "I pushed and forced and tried harder and harder and seemed to get nowhere or injured." What's happening? You are not natural anymore. You are too tense, too uncoordinated, too muscle-bound, too weak, or too hung-up in one way or another. You usually need help and time to learn how to do things right, and that takes patience.

The mastering of a foreign language, which takes most people a long time, can serve as an example. You set out by memorizing vocabulary and verb conjugations, and by working on simple phrases. But it's a long road before you can think and communicate without effort in a new language. Whether you are learning to play an instrument or to drop-volley in tennis, real mastery takes a very long time. We take weekend courses and seminars that promise to change our lives instantly. We turn to pills and magic cures that promise immediate gratification, but when we take an honest look at all these grasping efforts we are usually disappointed in the results.

Sport or exercise cannot be learned properly by imitating the quick, mechanized ways of our push-button society. Your body is not a machine. It is practically the only connection with nature you have left. If you develop it slowly and carefully through proper exercise, you can get the maximum return from a valuable resource. The body won't turn on like a television; it needs time to warm up and develop. If injured, it won't spring right back into action—it needs to be gently coaxed. If you take the time to become proficient at a sport or exercise program, you will have to learn patience along the way. The wishful expectation that big changes happen quickly is an invitation to disappointment. In our modern technological society of rapid external change, it is easy to forget that patience is probably one of the greatest assets you can ever possess.

## RELAXATION, EXERCISE, AND SLEEP

Each person's daily activity includes the invariable buildup of excess tension. Alleviating this tension is essential to your health. Unfortunately, it is not as easy to discharge this tension and relax as one might think.

Most people believe that they relax while they sleep. This is usually not the case. The body is only a little less tense during sleep than while awake. This is also true of resting, which is not necessarily relaxing, either. For instance, if you lie in bed for many days, you will probably find that your muscles have become very tight and stiff.

Exercise is very effective in taking the edge off of the daily buildup of tension, but it cannot solve the deeper problems of chronic excess tension. In fact, exercise is not necessarily relaxing, because some exercises actually increase muscular tension. It depends on what you do and how you do it.

Genuine relaxation can be attained through a balance of the right type of activity and rest. Some good exercises for relaxation are described in Chapter 6.

## HOW TO TAKE CARE OF YOUR BODY

If you are in good health generally, you will be able to pursue your sports activities safely, and you will play better. Health is an internal, day-to-day balance created by your style of living, and to be in good shape you must know how to care for yourself. Listed below are body-care techniques that are helpful in maintaining low levels of tension and high levels of health. They are useful in avoiding stiffness, fatigue, and tension, and can add to your general well-being. These techniques are passive, and do not require as much energy as exercising. Nonetheless, they do require some effort. Good health is in your hands. It requires initiative, knowledge, and some work. You will find the time and energy expended well worth it.

**Baths:** One of the most important, easiest, and most enjoyable body-care techniques is a nightly half-hour bath. (However, if you have heart trouble, you should check with your doctor first.) The water should be comfortably warm but not too hot, although tolerance to heat varies from person to person. The water should be pleasant to get into and not cause you to perspire while in the bath. Extreme heat perpetuates tension and shocks your system. A warm bath, on the other hand, draws tension from the body. The gentle buoyancy of the water has a relaxing effect, and clean skin breathes better because the pores are unclogged. Concentrate on relaxing your body while in the bath. Don't neglect your head. Submerge yourself several times so that only your eyes, nose, and mouth are above the water. Rub your skin firmly with a stiff brush or loofah sponge to stimulate circulation at the skin surface. Occasionally add two cups of sea salt or rock salt to your bath. The salt facilitates relaxation by increasing the tension-drawing effect of the water. If you've gone swimming both in oceans and in lakes, you may have noticed the effects of salt water on your body. The ocean salt water makes you feel pleasantly tired, whereas when you emerge from a fresh-water lake, you are usually invigorated.

**Whirlpool Baths:** Whirlpool baths accelerate the healing of most injuries and are excellent for your general health as well. A whirlpool usually looks like an oversized bathtub, with about six strong jets. These jets shoot the water into your body and around the tub with varying degrees of force. A whirlpool stimulates blood circulation, massaging the body with a very gentle hand, so to speak.

Whirlpools can be purchased for home use—it's good to have one if you can afford it. They are also commonly used in health clubs and hospitals. The optimal temperature for a whirlpool bath varies for different individuals. A problem in using one in a public facility is that the water temperature is often much too hot. As mentioned above, this can do more harm than good. If you use a whirlpool in a public facility, speak up and educate the people who run it. Take a whirlpool for fifteen to thirty minutes, depending on your preference.

**Shower Massage:** The shower massage is a showerhead pipe attachment that releases pulsating streams of water in speeds ranging from slow to fast, and it is an effective tool for relaxation. It is also good for sore muscles and helps increase blood circulation.

Use it as hard as you can take it in the fast-pulsating position. Direct it especially to the forehead, top and back of the head, neck, fingertips, hands, arms, down the full extent of the trunk, legs, feet, and even the toes, heels, and soles. Keep it on aching or fatigued areas for long periods of time.

**Sauna and Steam:** Both the sauna and the steam room can help you relax. The sauna is slightly more effective, especially for those who tend to be claustrophobic. (However, if you have heart trouble, check with your doctor as a precautionary measure.) In a sauna, dry heat makes you perspire. Thus, the moisture comes from inside the body. In a steam room, the moisture is part perspiration and part condensed steam. In either case, you can sit, lie flat, or elevate your legs (see below). Be sure to breathe deeply. Your first exposures to sauna and steam should be brief. Begin with two- to five-minute sessions and slowly increase exposure to a maximum of twenty to thirty minutes. Exposure to these types of heat is relaxing and beneficial, but build your tolerance for them slowly. A bucket of cold water and a face cloth to squeeze over your head can help prevent headache. If you're feeling claustrophobic, place the wet face cloth over your face and breathe through it. However, if the experience becomes too unpleasant, leave immediately and take a cool shower. You can go back and forth repeatedly between a cool shower and a sauna or steam room.

**Elevating the Legs:** Tension in the legs can be alleviated by lying on the back on the floor and resting the legs against a wall at a 45-degree angle, or resting the lower legs on a chair, for five to ten minutes once or twice a day. Be sure not to lock the knees and to keep them slightly bent.

When you are standing, your blood must defy gravity to return to your heart. By elevating your legs, you help your blood circulation, as well as relaxing certain parts of your nervous system. It is like giving your legs an hour of sleep. This exercise is especially helpful if you

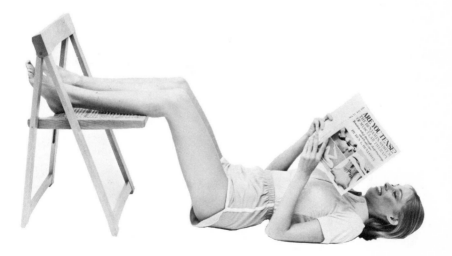

spend a good deal of time on your feet, since it encourages blood circulation in the legs. While elevating your legs, you can read, talk on the phone, or do anything you like. (If you have a heart condition, however, check with your doctor, since this exercise is recommended for some heart conditions but is dangerous for others.)

**Chair and Table Heights:** If you spend a lot of time sitting in one particular chair or using a certain table, either at home or in the office, you should be aware of the fact that their dimensions may effect your body in many ways. The best kind of chair provides a few inches of padding on a firm foundation and allows your feet to rest firmly on the ground. It should be of a height that permits your legs to slope down slightly from the hip to the knee, with the lower leg perpendicular to the floor. Different people require chairs of varying heights. The proper height is generally the distance from the bottom of your heel to the

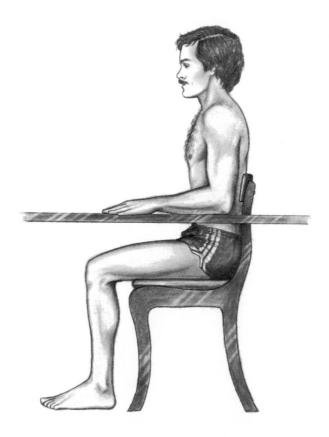

back of your knee when you are in a sitting position. A low chair is bad for the lower back; it tips the pelvis backward. A chair that is too high is not as dangerous, although it can hamper circulation from the knees down. The depth of the chair should match the distance from behind the knee to the back of the hip. A shallow chair is not harmful, but one that is too deep encourages you to lean back and slump your lower back.*

Tables and desks that are too high force you to raise your shoulders. If they are too low, you'll lean over and strain your lower back. The proper height for a table or desk depends on the length of your trunk and arms. If the table comes up to your elbow when you are sitting with arms bent, it is the proper height. Before deciding upon your table or desk height, be sure your chair height is correct. Propping your feet up when you sit at a desk may feel good, but it adds strain and pressure to your lower back. Keep your feet on the ground.

**Shoes:** The most healthful and comfortable shoes are those that are shaped like the foot. They should be moderately squared off at the toes. If the shoes have pointed toes that squeeze the feet, the toes will be pushed together and the feet will become tense. If you observe people's feet at the beach, you'll see many sets of toes jammed together from too-narrow shoes or hammered down from shoes that are too short.

Platform shoes are especially dangerous and totally unnatural. The Association of Podiatrists has issued a statement on the frequency of accidents due to platform shoes. Shoes with very high heels are bad for both the feet and the legs, since they place them at unnatural angles. Similarly, the popular new shoes with the heel lower than the toe are also extremely destructive for most people. They shift the weight unnaturally back to the heel and place stress on the Achilles tendon, calf muscles, and lower back. If you try to run in negative-heel shoes, you probably will feel pain in your legs. A low heel, however, does no damage. If you have very short Achilles tendons, you might do well to exercise with sponge lifts in the heels of your shoes. This will reduce stress on the tendons.

---

* In sitting it is important to maintain the natural forward curve in your lower back. Those with lower back problems should place a little pillow in the small of their backs. Special Posture Curve[tm] Lumbar Cushions are available from R.T.I., P.O. Box 1045, New York, N.Y. 10025.

Sneakers and soft shoes are best, since man was meant to walk on the soft earth. Shoes shouldn't hold you up; muscles should do that job. A rule of thumb might be: The less constricting and softer the shoe, the better. Choose a shoe that allows the foot to bend in any direction and provides complete freedom of movement. As the hardness of the ground increases, so should the softness of our shoes. If the sole is too hard, try two Dr. Scholl's inner soles, sized to the length of your foot, in each shoe.

**Swimming:** Swimming is an excellent adjunct to any exercise program. It is the best exercise because it uses almost every muscle in the body and increases respiration. Moreover, the body is weightless in water and therefore is unlikely to be injured. And water is, as we have seen, relaxing and therapeutic.

When I say swim to relax, I don't mean competitive swimming. Have a good time. Float a little, do a few laps, kick on your back, on your stomach, submerge your body in deep water, and stretch in all directions. If you're feeling creative, do an underwater dance. The breast stroke is especially good exercise because it uses all muscles equally. Swimming daily or two to three times a week will do wonders, but if you have lower back problems, avoid diving.

## A CLOSING NOTE ON COMMON SENSE

If you push yourself beyond your limit, you might get hurt. Play as long as you should, not for every second of the time you paid for the court. Simple good sense, yes, but most don't follow it. It's like going out to dinner, getting a lousy meal, and eating it because it cost so much, then getting sick and feeling bad for the rest of the evening.

Know how long you can exercise and remain feeling good and not get sore the next day. Know what sports and exercises you can't do without hurting yourself because of your bad knee, old lower back injury, or weak ankles. If you have deteriorating cartilage in your knee, running is out but swimming is in. If you tend to get lower back pain, deep back bends are out and so is the cobra in yoga, but tai chi is fine. If you have ankles that are very unstable and sprain easily, ice skating is out, but running in place or a good ballet class might make you stronger.

Know your heart and its endurance. Your heart is a muscle, too. Keep your heart running strong, but don't strain it. If you get chest pain when you run, it may be as simple as a stitch spasm of the diaphragm but it might be the warning of a heart attack.

Nausea during exercise or sport with any regularity could mean a variety of things from bad food to a brain tumor. That's one thing you should look into. If you get dizzy regularly when active you might just breathe poorly or you might have TB.

If you get little muscular and joint pains or aches in your body that move from place to place all the time, it's most probably accumulated muscular tension, but it might also be the beginnings of rheumatoid arthritis, so see your doctor to make sure.

Occasional little twinges of sharp pain in your lower back or down the back of your thigh may be the beginnings of a kidney disease, disc trouble, or sciatica from chronic tension, poor posture, or unevenly developed muscle balance and strength. You may have time to change it if you listen and seek the appropriate help. You may be doing exercises that are bad for your body or you may be using muscles only on one side (as in tennis) and this might not be so good for your scoliosis (sideways curve of the spine) unless you do special exercises to balance things out.

The list of dos and don'ts is as long as our capacity for endless variation, creativity, and stupidity. Let these truisms help you make contact with your own needs. Make your own list of dos and dont's, and may you have the strength and intelligence to follow your list.

# 3

# WARM-UP!
# THE MISSING LINK
# IN EXERCISE

Warming up. We hear about it, we seldom do it, we hardly understand it at all. Warming up is like tuning a fine instrument. It allows your body to respond to your commands quicker and easier. It increases your body's capacity for sustained exercise and insures that many injuries will not occur.

You don't set out on an extended journey without first preparing your car for the trip. You check the oil, the brakes, the tires, even get it tuned up and lubricated to make sure that it won't break down somewhere along the way. But when it comes to our own bodies, we often subject them to severe physical stress without adequately preparing them. And they break down, too.

What happens when you don't warm up? Torn or pulled muscles, sprained ankles, back spasms, sciatica, torn cartilage, shin splints are just a few of the injuries that can result. Most of these injuries can be avoided. A body that's been warmed up is like a resilient green twig: It can absorb stress and remain supple. Without warming up, the body is like a dry stick, breaking under pressure.

Professional athletes recognize the importance of warming up before any sports or exercise activity and never neglect to do so from five to fifteen minutes before a game. They know it's important even though they often don't warm up in the best possible way. Whether it's an activity as calm as golf or as vigorous as tennis, basketball, or a dance class, a warm-up is well worth the time and energy, and it doesn't take much of either. Generally, warming up should take from ten to fifteen minutes. In very warm weather, six to seven minutes can be enough. But when it's extremely cold, it might take slightly longer.

## WARMING UP PHYSIOLOGICALLY PREPARES THE BODY FOR THE INCREASED STRESS OF EXERCISE

**Blood Supply and Muscles:** Warming up actually means making your body heat increase. When the nutrients in your body are used it's like a furnace burning fuel for energy: Heat is produced as a by-product. This heat is then distributed throughout your body by the system of blood circulation. It's like the boiler in your basement heating water that is circulated through your radiators. The blood literally carries the heat around your body. In a sense you begin to steam-heat your muscles, making them warm and more flexible. When you begin to move with a little more vigor, you burn more fuel and increase the temperature of your blood, which then heats your muscles. Increased blood flow in turn carries more nutrients and supplies additional oxygen, both of which are needed by the muscles to sustain vigorous exercise. Enlarged by the additional blood, the muscles become more resilient and flexible, just as a dry sponge does when it absorbs water. Nerve impulses travel faster and more efficiently through warmed and more fluid tissues. In addition, warmed-up muscles are more responsive to these impulses. Tense muscles affect blood circulation in a way similar to that in which standing on a hose affects water flow. If you suffer from excess tension, your body needs to work harder to warm up. So give yourself more time to warm up.

**Breathing:** Breathing supplies your body with oxygen, which ignites the fire to burn your fuel. It is important to increase your breathing rate gradually and not suddenly in order to supply the increased demand for oxygen. Without gradually preparing the respiratory system, we tire very quickly and often end up panting after a few minutes of vigorous exercise. The most important and neglected part of respiration is exhaling. Most people do not exhale fully; they keep a residual volume of used air which stagnates in the bottom of their lungs. Deep, regular breathing during exercise is extremely important. Fatigue is often caused by shallow breathing or by partially holding your breath during exercise. Warming up the diaphragm by slowly increasing your breathing rate and paying attention to how you breathe can set the tone for more consistent breathing during more vigorous exercise. Having a warmed-up diaphragm helps you to avoid premature fatigue and stitch pain.

**The Heart:** The heart is a muscle and, therefore, needs additional blood and nutrients to increase its capacity for the harder and faster pumping which is needed during vigorous activity. The heart muscle may suffer great stress if it doesn't readjust its internal circulation gradually. Warming up prepares the muscles of the heart for the exercise or sport to come in the same way that it prepares other muscles.

**The Joints:** Joints are bathed in a special fluid called synovial fluid, which acts as oil would in a hinge. As we use a joint the body produces more synovial fluid to increase the lubrication and reduce friction. This slowly accelerates as the stress and vigor of joint movement increases. If stress increases too suddenly or too quickly, fluid production lags behind and joint injury is much more likely to occur. Preparing the joints as the first part of any warm-up program is an important and often neglected step in preparation for sports or exercise.

## GENERAL PRINCIPLES

Warming up involves the gradual and coordinated preparation of the muscles, joints, lungs, and heart. Effective warm-up exercises consist exclusively of light to moderate strength-building activities. They aren't very strenuous and you should never have to strain while doing them. Warm-ups should begin while lying on the floor because this will enable you to gradually warm up the ankle, knee, and hip joints before they have the body's full weight going through them. Stretching exercises physiologically do *not* warm you up because warming up requires active muscle contraction, while stretching involves only lengthening and releasing muscles.

When you warm up there are several things to take into account: (1) what kind of activity you are getting ready for; (2) at what intensity you will begin it; (3) what part of the body is most intensively used; (4) what your physical limitations are. Let's say you are going to play tennis, that you will begin by playing doubles, and that it's your custom to volley for a long time before getting into the game. For this you need to warm up your whole body and to spend extra time on warming your upper body, especially your arm. On the other hand, if you're going to play singles and move quickly into a fast game, but you tend to have trouble with your knees, you should do a general warm-up, an upper-lower body combination warm-up, and then some special exercises for your legs and especially for your knees to get them ready for action. Chapter 4 explains the various warm-up programs in detail, Chapter 5 will help to pinpoint your body's weaknesses, and Chapter 10 gives advice on warming up for your particular sport.

Another factor is the weather. In the summer, the muscles of the body are all in a more expanded state naturally and tend to warm up quite easily. In the winter, even if you exercise indoors, the muscles are in a slightly more contracted state and take a little more time and patience. This is very literal. Some people's shoe sizes change as much as a half inch from summer to winter.

Always spend extra time warming up a part of your body that has a tendency to be injured or tense. It's like taking out a little insurance. Warming up cannot *guarantee* that you will not be injured, but it will greatly decrease the likelihood of injury. You will enter your sport or exercise with all your faculties at your disposal. Your muscles will be juiced up, your joints will be as lubricated as possible to lessen friction, your heart will be ready to supply you with enough oxygen, and your body and mind will be hot and ready to go.

## WARMING DOWN

After playing, it is very important to allow your body to slow down gradually. Sitting down immediately after vigorous exercise is not good for your body. Some people even become faint due to a too abrupt cessation of activity. Your heart is pumping lots of blood and you have to allow it to slow down over a two- to five-minute period, depending on the vigor of your previous activity and your physical condition. Stand, walk, or do an easy, slow jog to warm down. We know enough to walk horses to readjust their breathing rates; we should apply the same horse sense to people.

# 4

# THE BENJAMIN WARM-UP
# PROGRAM

Warming up isn't magic. You must do the activity that you're warming up for correctly. You must be aware of your limitations and know how to move. Such awareness and knowledge along with the right warm-ups goes a long way toward insuring safety during any strenuous exercise or activity.

Although the warm-up exercises in this chapter are simple and easy to do, don't underestimate their effectiveness. You shouldn't pant or strain during any of these exercises. If any of them cause you pain or even slight discomfort, your body is telling you that something is wrong. Stop and try to find out what's going on. If you are stiff or sore for any reason, go easy and skip any exercises which cause you discomfort. Never push through any of these exercises; eliminate them if they hurt.

These warm-ups get your body ready in a progressive, logical order. They slowly increase the demand on your joints, muscles, and respiratory and circulatory systems. A few of the last exercises are more vigorous in order to increase your heart rate. Don't push or move through them too quickly. Make sure you *breathe* gently and easily *during* every exercise.

## CREATING YOUR WARM-UP PROGRAM

Most athletic and exercise activities require you to use your entire body in some way; many, however, accent the upper or lower body. The upper body is primary in such activities as rowing or bowling, the lower body in such sports as running and skiing. I have organized the warm-up exercises into the following sections:

*The General Body Warm-up*: This series should be done before all sports or exercise or vigorous activities.

*The Lower-Body Warm-up*: This should be added to the general body warm-up exercises for running, skiing, ice skating, roller skating, hiking, bicycling, basketball, soccer, and football.

*The Upper-Body Warm-up*: This should be added to the general body warm-up for golf, rowing, bowling, wrestling, boxing, canoeing, sailing, archery, and kayaking.

*The Upper-Lower Combination Warm-up*: This combines the exercises from the previous two sets to best prepare you for the activities that place a relatively equal demand on both the upper and lower segments of the body. Do this series after the general body warm-up for tennis, baseball, softball, gymnastics, volleyball, hockey, handball, squash, racquetball, paddleball, platform tennis, cross-country skiing, badminton, karate, aikido, judo, fencing, and water skiing.

*The Dance Warm-up*: Add this slightly different combination to the general body warm-up before dance and exercise classes.

If an area of your body needs extra warming up, work with it a little longer or return to it more frequently. You can also add some of the minor strength-building exercises (Chapter 8) to your warm-up if you are returning from inactivity or recovering from an injury.

A summary listing the different series of warm-ups can be found on page 94.

## REPETITION

It's important to avoid too much repetition during the warm-ups. The body resists repetition. Even a terrific meal becomes tiresome after several days. Likewise, when you do the same exercise over and over, the body's circuits overload and you get fatigued.

Varying the movements is essential, because it allows some muscles to rest while others are in use. If you hold one arm straight out to the side for five minutes, the muscle will fatigue, your arm will tire and begin to hurt. This is because contraction was sustained for too long, which depletes both the oxygen and energy. On the other hand, if you alternate holding your arm out for sixty seconds, and then resting for thirty, you could hold it up for an accumulated period of half an hour or more. The rest periods allow the body time to recuperate.

A third possibility is to keep the arm moving, swinging it from side to side, up and down in various patterns. The movement, momentum, and variation take weight off the muscle, allowing it to recuperate. In addition, the fluid movement involves many more muscles of the back and shoulder area. This pumps extra blood, oxygen, and energy into the arm. So keep alternating sides, and change the exercises frequently after about five or six repetitions.

## WHERE TO WARM UP

If you warm up at home, select a room with a nice rug or spread a blanket or towel out on the floor. Make sure there is enough space for you to lie on your back and move your arms and legs in all directions without bumping into anything. It's preferable to keep the room comfortably warm. If you are outside, a flat grassy area is best.

If you have a bony sacrum (the bone at the base of the spine between the hips), keep a small pillow or towel on hand. The sacrum sometimes needs to be cushioned when your legs are in the air.

If you like music, warm up or exercise to anything from Bach to the Beatles. Make warming-up and exercising as enjoyable as you can.

## WHAT TO WEAR

Wear loose-fitting clothes, because they're easier to move in. Socks are okay, but take off your shoes if you can. I warm up in my running clothes so I can run out the door and right into the park.

## THE WARM-UP TRICK

There is a trick to cut your warm-up time almost in half. It's also useful if your body is quite tense and generally stiff, and you find it hard to get warmed-up. Soak in a *warm* bath for five or six minutes directly before you begin your warm-up. This increases blood circulation and "cooks" the muscles. They will respond faster because the bath makes them more pliable.

## DEFINITIONS

To clarify a few working definitions: When I mention the word *replace* in describing an exercise, I mean return to your original position. *Extend* means to straighten your leg an inch or two off the floor from a starting position lying on your back. *A complete set* means to perform the movements on both the right and left sides.

## THE GENERAL BODY WARM-UP

# 1.

### Breathing

To begin, lie down on your back and relax. Concentrate on deepening your breathing. Without pushing or forcing, take ten to fifteen breaths. Make sure that your exhales are a little longer than your inhales. Don't puff your chest up or push your abdomen out, but rather let your breathing ebb and flow easily like the rhythm of an ocean. The lower chest and upper abdomen should rise and fall simultaneously, if you aren't forcing your breathing. Breathe through an open mouth in order to prevent clenching your jaw and throat. Breathing in this manner is the first step toward relaxation as well as good preparation for any movement activity.

*We will start from the bottom and work our way up.*

# 2.

### Toe Flexion

While remaining in the lying position, begin by flexing and extending your toes. Concentrate on a continuous action rather than stopping at each position. Flex and extend the toes as fully as you can without moving the ankle joint. Do ten to fifteen flexion-extension sets without forcing.

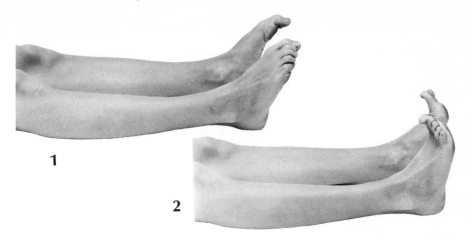

1

2

This exercise increases synovial-fluid production in the toe joints, warms up the nineteen muscles of the foot, and begins to work the muscles in the lower leg which move the toes.

*Next, we warm up both the ankle joint and the muscles of the lower leg.*

## 3.

### Ankle Circles

Rotate the foot to its limit in a wide circle, either lying flat or with your leg in the air as in Exercise 4. Move each foot in one direction for a while, and then in the other. Circle your ankles either separately or together. Remember not to do any one exercise for too long a period of time.

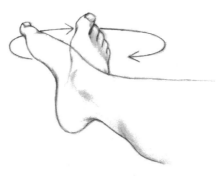

## 4.

## Ankle Flexion

Bend your knees toward your chest and place your hands on top of your knees, suspending your legs in the air. You can also cross one leg over the other. Ankle flexion can either be done with one foot at a time or with both feet simultaneously. Point and flex your feet slowly. Try not to stop at any point during the exercise. Move continually and without a lot of force.

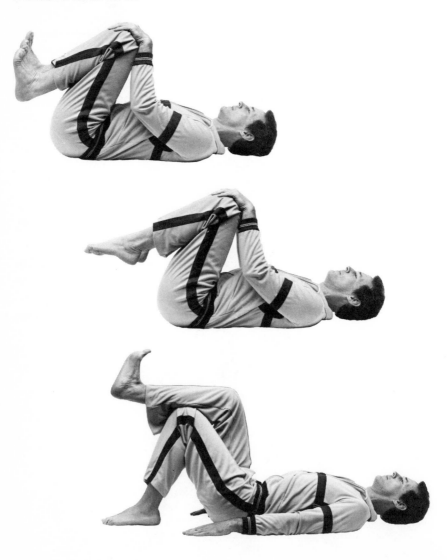

Ankle Circles and Ankle Flexion stimulate synovial fluid production in the ankle joint. In addition, these exercises warm up those muscles of the lower leg that control extension, flexion, and the side-to-side movements of the foot. The circulation of this area is now increasing as a greater volume of blood is being moved through the legs.

## 5.

### Foot-Shaking

Bend your knees toward your chest and lift your legs in the air, keeping your knees slightly bent. Shake your feet and legs forcefully for about thirty to forty seconds. Allow your ankles to flop and your legs to be loose like jelly. It is important to keep breathing throughout this exercise. It's easy to forget and hold your breath, thus tightening your abdomen.

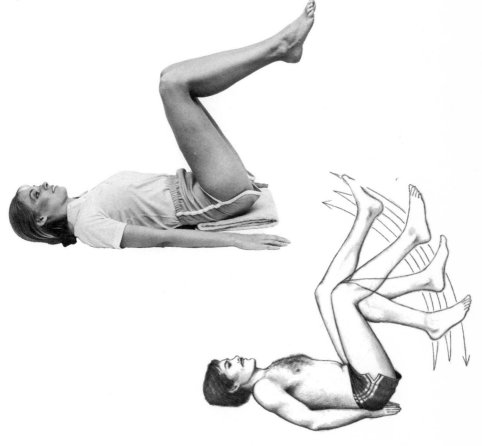

The weight of your legs should be easily balanced over your pelvis or abdomen. This prevents you from straining the lower back and abdominal muscles. If it is difficult to keep your legs up, take the *sacral guard position* by placing a folded bath towel under your buttocks or by placing your hands flat on the floor under your lower spine as shown. If this does not give you enough height, cross your hands over one another for more support. Use the sacral guard position whenever you need to in the exercises that follow. This position accomplishes two goals: (1) raises the bony, often unpadded, sacral bone slightly off the ground so that it doesn't grind into the floor; (2) brings the weight of the legs over the chest in order to minimize the stress on the abdominal and lower back muscles.

Never lift both legs at once while keeping them straight. This can cause strain and tension in the lower back and abdomen, especially if you're not warmed up. When lifting your legs up, always bend your knees toward your chest first.

Foot-shaking relaxes the muscles of the foot and lower leg. At the same time it begins gently to warm up the muscles of the thigh, and slightly increases the synovial fluid production in the knees and hip joints.

*When you begin your warm-up, do the exercises in the order given, then do them again using a random sequence for the first five exercises if you wish. Do not repeat the action of any one of these exercises more than eight times in a row. It is best if you do a few of one, go on to another, do it a few times, come back to the first, and continue changing.*

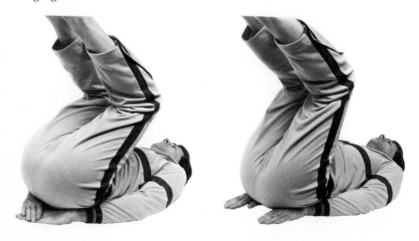

## 6.

The parts of Exercises 6 and 8 gradually increase in difficulty and are therefore more demanding on your body. Throughout this section, lying on your back, knees bent and feet flat on the floor as shown, will be referred to as *the basic position*.

### 6A.
### The Knee-to-Chest

While lying in the basic position, raise one knee toward your chest as far as it will go without straining or lifting the back of the pelvis off the floor. Then return your leg to the basic position. If you like, occasionally grasp your knee and pull it slightly farther toward your chest. Alternating right and left legs, do four or five sets slowly.

The Basic Position

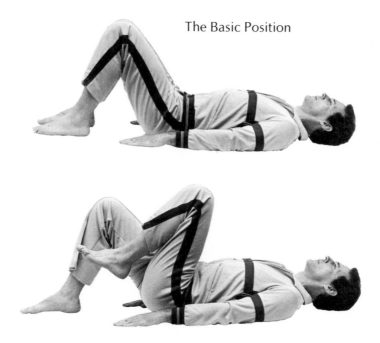

6B.
## The Knee-to-Chest, with a Foot Throw

This is a modification of the previous exercise. Instead of leading with your knee, lead with your toes as though you were gently tossing your foot over your head in a big arc. Do this in one motion. At the high point of the movement you should be able to see your toes. Also, make sure to keep the back of your pelvis on the floor. Don't kick or force the movement. Alternate using the right and left legs. Make sure to replace one foot on the floor before lifting the other. Do four or five sets, alternating right and left legs.

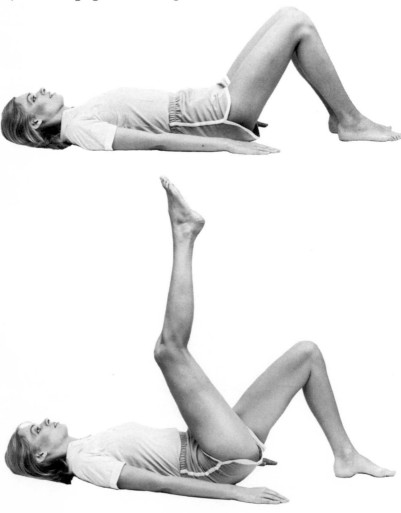

6C.
## Chest, Extend, Chest, Replace

This exercise begins in the basic position and has four parts. First, lift one knee to your chest. Second, extend the leg so that it's one or two inches above the ground. Third, bring it back to your chest, and fourth, return it to the basic position. Be sure to alternate your legs. Do four or five sets.

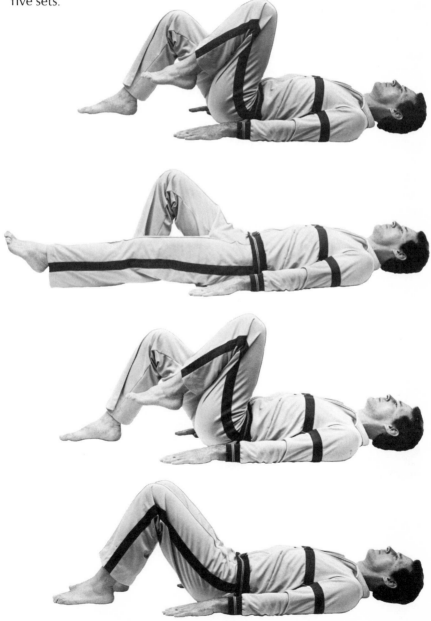

All parts of Exercise 6 warm up the muscles of the front thigh, increase fluid production in the hip joint, and start the warm-up of the lower back and abdomen. In addition, they generally increase blood circulation in the pelvic area.

## 7.
### The Pelvic Tilt and Lift

Once again, lie in the basic position. Tilt your pelvis forward so that your lower back touches the floor. Keeping the tilt, slowly lift your pelvis 2 or 3 inches off the ground. Now gently lower it to the floor. Do this eight or ten times, resting a moment between each one.

To do this exercise, you don't have to contract your abdominal or buttock muscles noticeably, for most of the work should be done by deep muscles, which are difficult to feel. Try to do the tilting by pressing your feet into the ground and exhaling. Do this exercise very slowly, and be careful not to hold your breath. This is to allow the body a recovery from the previous exercise, in preparation for the next one, which requires more exertion. Remember to breathe!

The Pelvic Tilt and Lift warms up the muscles at the back of the thigh and the deep muscles of the abdomen. Additionally, it lengthens and helps to release some tension in the lower-back area.

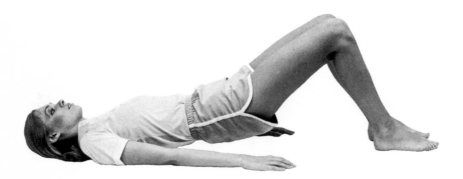

8.

## Chest, Extend, Lift, Replace

**8A.** Lying in the basic position, bring your knee to your chest. Now extend one leg so that it's straight, and an inch or two above the floor. Lift the leg straight up in the air toward the ceiling, then return it to your original position. Don't forcefully kick the leg when you lift it. Keep your feet relaxed for the first set.

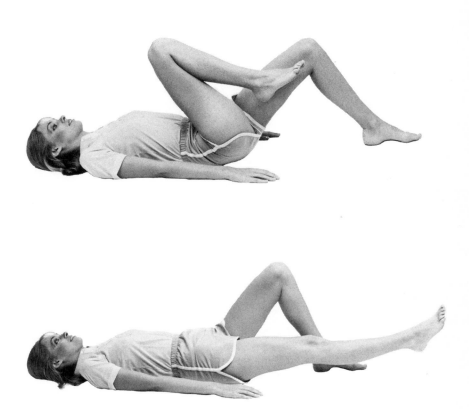

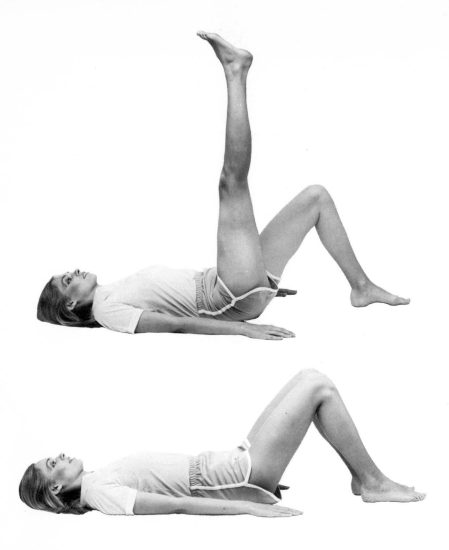

After you've alternated legs six to eight times, flex the foot as you go from the first to the second position and try it again.

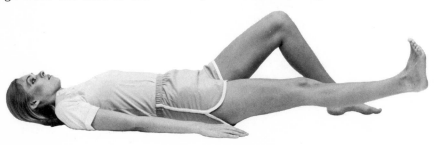

**8B.** Repeat Exercise 8A, modifying the lift. Instead of lifting your leg toward the ceiling, let it open up and out toward the wall, forming a 45-degree angle with the floor. Do this version six to eight times with a relaxed foot, alternating legs, and then six to eight times going into flexion as you extend the leg.

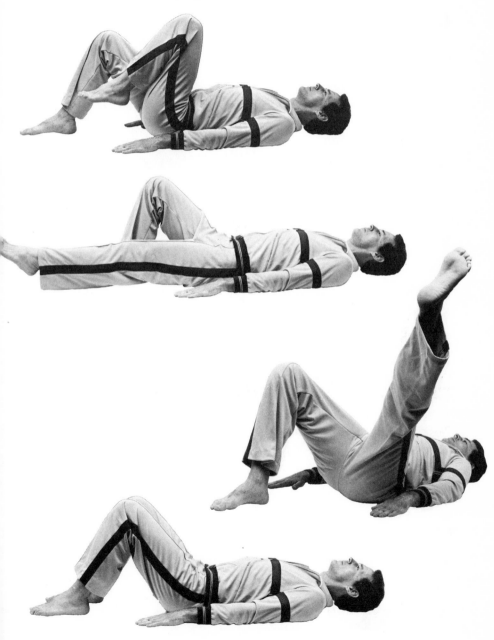

**8C.** In this variation, do the four beats, this time lifting the leg out to the side as close to the floor as you can without straining or allowing the opposite side of the pelvis to come off the floor. Then return it to the basic position. Alternate legs with and without the foot flexed.

These exercises lubricate the knee and hip joints, and warm up the muscles of the abdomen, lower back, pelvis, and legs, especially the thighs.

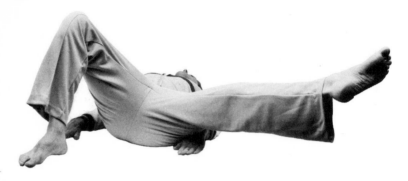

## 9.

### Chest, Circle Out, Extend, Replace

**9A.** Starting in the basic position, bring your right knee to your chest. Keeping your back on the floor and your knee bent, open your right leg to the side as far as it will go. Now extend your leg downward as you draw it back in line with your body to the familiar extended position two to three inches off the floor. Then return your right leg to the basic position. Now try it with the left leg.

As you learn this exercise, imagine your knee drawing a curved arc in space as it opens to the side and swings down to the extended position. Once you have the movement fluid and easy try doing two or three continuous loops with the right leg before replacing it in the basic position and switching to the left.

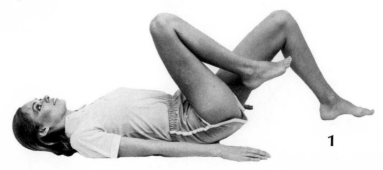

1

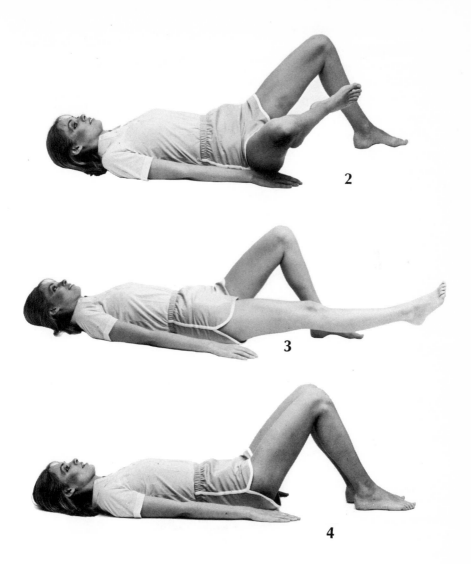

2

3

4

**9B.** This time reverse the movement so that the knee circles in the opposite direction. Begin with one knee in the basic position, and your working leg extended resting on the floor. Lift the knee of the extended leg to the side, loop it around up toward your chest, and place it back down onto the floor. Once you've learned this, do two to three loops in succession without letting the leg touch the floor.

These exercises warm up the muscles of the inner and outer thigh, the lower back, the abdomen, and the waist. They also warm up the muscles surrounding the hip joint.

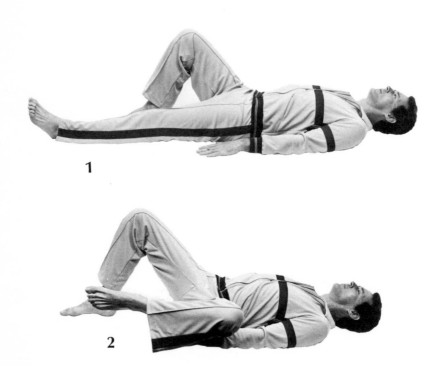

**1**

**2**

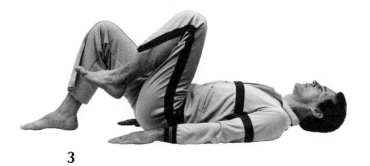

3

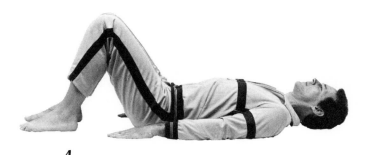

4

## 10.

### The Lower-Back Twist

Lie in the basic position with your arms extended out to the side below shoulder level, palms down. Lower both knees to the left, allowing your right knee to move up toward your left elbow as it gets closer to the floor. Once you've gone as far as you can without straining, try to relax into the twist. Depending on your natural flexibility, you can place your knee anywhere from 2 inches to 2 feet below your left elbow. Your right arm will probably raise up off the floor. Do not force it down. Try to relax and release the shoulder and arm by breathing. If your arm or shoulder is too uncomfortable, lower your arm closer to your side or drape it across your ribs.

Remain in this position long enough to take a few deep breaths. Now, move back through the basic position and do the same on the opposite side. After you've done this two to three times on each side, proceed, changing from side to side without the rests and at a moderate tempo. Do this only five or six times on each side. Be sure not to hold your breath.

This exercise warms up the rotating muscles of the lower and mid-back as well as the muscles of the thigh.

*After you have gone through these exercises once in order you can create your own random sequence with Exercises 6 through 10. Do only four or five of each exercise and then move on to the next. It's all right to do each of these exercises a total of fifteen to twenty times if you keep mixing up the sequence. The principle to keep in mind here is to alternate to avoid fatiguing any one set of muscles. This is what happens if you push them too far too quickly, or work them too long.*

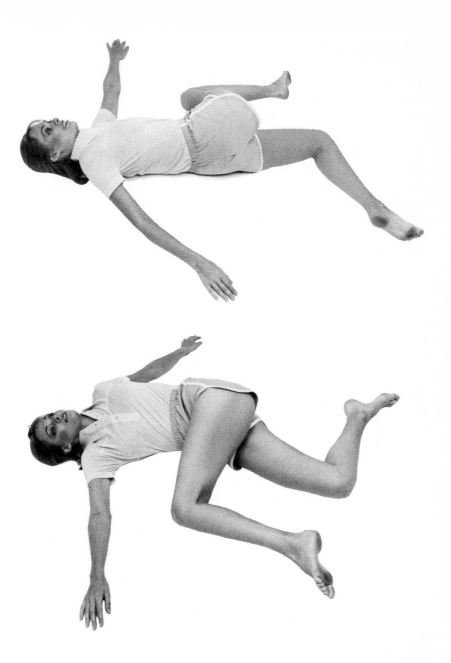

## 11.

### The Bicycle

To help center the weight of your legs over your chest, cross your hands in the sacral guard position (see Exercise 5) and place them under your sacrum at the lower end of your spine.

First, bend your knees up toward your chest. Now begin making a bicycle action toward the sky or ceiling, as the case may be. Your feet should neither be relaxed nor tightly flexed, but kept in a slightly flexed position. Reach upward with the soles of your feet each time your leg straightens in the air. Be absolutely sure to keep breathing throughout this exercise. It's easy to tighten your breath on this one, because you are using your abdominal muscles. A good way to insure that you are breathing properly is to keep your mouth open and make a gentle "ah" sound as you do it.

Try to have your feet above your chest, rather than over your pelvis. This will reduce stress on the abdomen.

The Bicycle should be done at a moderate to vigorous tempo. Bicycle for eight to ten seconds, rest for a moment, and then try it again for a bit longer. Repeat this two to three times.

The Bicycle exercise steps up your cardiovascular and respiratory systems. It also helps to integrate coordinated movement, and warms up the back, abdomen, thighs, shins, and hip muscles.

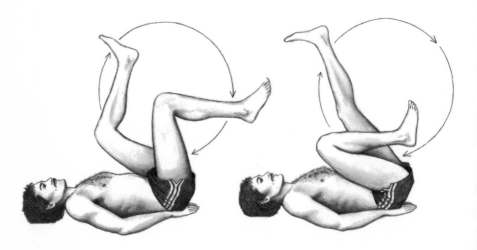

Now it's time to stand up. Roll onto your side, push yourself up to a sitting position, and stand up. This is always a safe way to rise from a supine position. It reduces the strain on the front of the neck and abdominal muscles as well as on the muscles of the lower back.

During all of the remaining exercises in this section, stand up with your feet parallel, about four to six inches apart. Check as frequently as necessary to make sure that they remain parallel. This is the most efficient position for standing. If it makes you uncomfortable, approximate it as much as you can without discomfort.

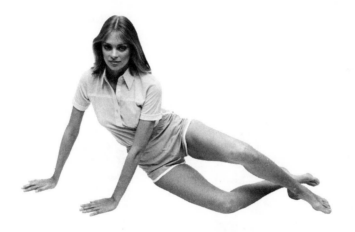

## 12.

### The Sky Reach

In the standing position, raise both arms straight above your head. Now alternate, reaching one arm at a time up toward the sky. Try to reach not only with the arm and hand, but from your waist. Gaze slightly upward, if you can do so with your neck relaxed. Do eight to ten reaches, alternating hands. Rest for a moment, and then do it again. Make sure that you don't hold your breath.

The Sky Reach warms up the muscles of the upper arm, the shoulder, the upper back, the waist, and even the lower back.

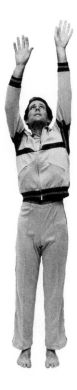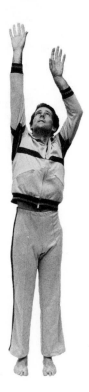

## 13.

### The Side Reach

Stand with your feet parallel, about 12 inches apart, distributing your weight evenly on both legs. Extend your arms directly to the sides at shoulder height. Now reach sideways out toward the wall with your right hand, only allowing the movement to occur in the upper body. When you've reached as far as you can, repeat with the left hand. Do not bend to the side. Do eight to ten right-left sets of this exercise.

The Side Reach warms up the muscles of the lower back and waist.

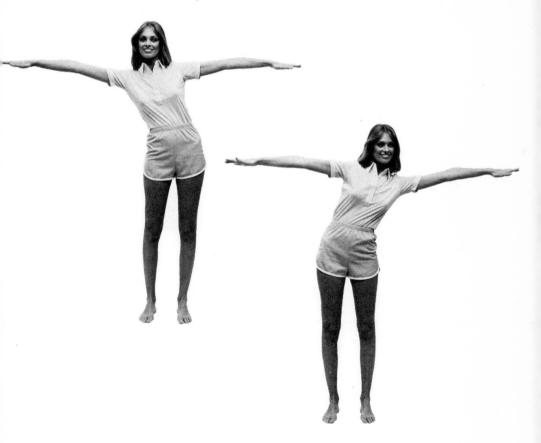

## 14.

### Shoulder Rolls

Roll your shoulders in a circular motion to their extreme range—up, back, down, and around. Make it a smooth circle, and breathe as you do it. Now reverse it, going up, forward, down, and back. You can roll both shoulders simultaneously or alternate them. Do eight or ten rolls in each direction.

This exercise warms up the muscles of the shoulders and upper back.

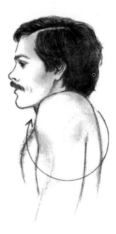

## 15.

### The Shoulder Drop

Remaining in the standing position, raise your shoulders toward your ears as high as you can. Then let them drop suddenly, allowing gravity to bring them down. Inhale when you raise the shoulders, and exhale as you drop them. This exercise should be done ten to fifteen times slowly, followed by ten to fifteen times quickly.

The Shoulder Drop warms up the muscles of the shoulders and upper back. It is additionally beneficial because it releases tension in the neck, shoulders, and upper-back area.

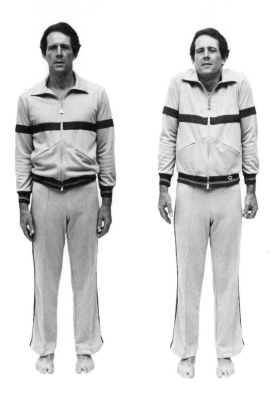

## 16.

### Hand-Shaking

Hold both hands in front of your chest and shake them rather vigorously. Keep shaking them as you slowly and gradually move your arms out to the sides, above your head, and then down again. Complete three or four of these circular movements. Remember to move the arms slowly, but shake your hands energetically.

This exercise warms up and helps relax the muscles of the hands, arms, and shoulders. It also works to lubricate the wrist joints and increase the circulation in the arm and shoulder area.

## 17.

### The Head Compass

From the standing position, slowly lower your head down toward your chest until you see the floor beneath you. Now, only going as far back as you comfortably can, raise your head and look at the sky. Do three to four sets of this front-back movement. Always keep your head in control; never drop or thrust it. Now, without moving your shoulders, turn your head as far as you can to one side, and then to the other. Never strain or push it. As your head moves, focus your eyes and look at the surroundings. This helps to keep the head and neck active so that you don't drop the weight of the head. Now, keep your gaze straight in front of you and tilt your head sideways by bringing your ear toward your shoulder. Do three or four left-right turn and tilt movements. Remember to focus your eyes and to breathe while doing these movements.

The neck is a very sensitive area. If any of these movements are difficult and cause you any discomfort, omit them from your warm-up program.

The Head Compass warms up the muscles of the neck and shoulders.

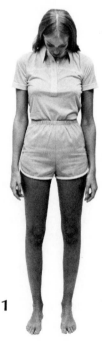
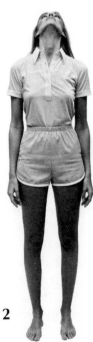

1                    2

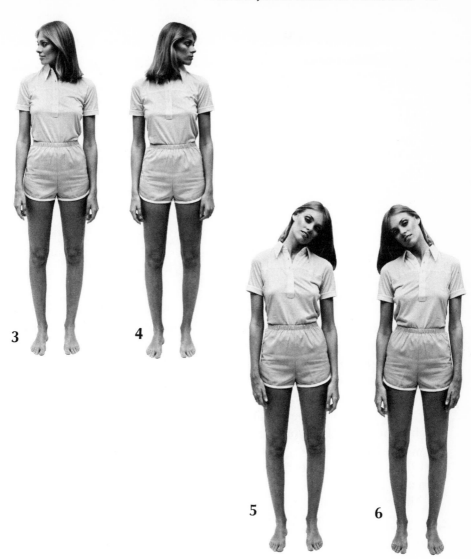

3   4   5   6

**Time Involved in the General Body Warm-up:** Once you've learned this segment of the warm-up, it should take you about six to eight minutes. However, it will initially take a bit longer until the exercises are familiar. Take the time to learn them thoroughly. Refer to the summary on page 94 when you're actually doing them.

## THE LOWER-BODY WARM-UP

### The Intermission Shake-out

Hold one foot a few inches off the ground and shake it and your leg for ten to twenty seconds. Now do this with the other foot. After doing this a few times, continue with your exercises. Do the shake-out any time that you feel like it during the lower-body warm-up to give your body a momentary breather.

## 1.

### The Knee Bend and Raise

Hold onto something sturdy and a little above waist level for balance and stand with your feet parallel about two or three inches apart. Keep your back erect and slowly bend your knees as much as you can without raising your heels off the floor. Don't push or force. Now, simultaneously straighten your legs and rise up onto the balls of your feet. Return to the starting position. Be sure to hold something high enough so that you can remain upright. Do this exercise very slowly eight or ten times. If your legs shake slightly as you come down off the balls of your feet, start with just a few of them to build up to ten over a week or two.

This exercise warms up all the muscles of the legs and feet in addition to increasing fluid secretions in the ankle and knee joints.

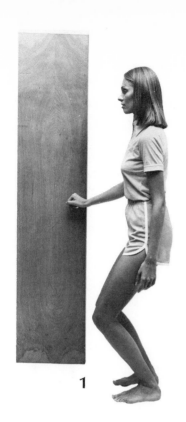

1

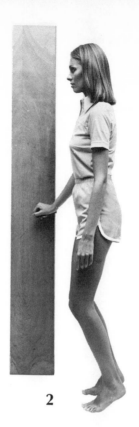

3

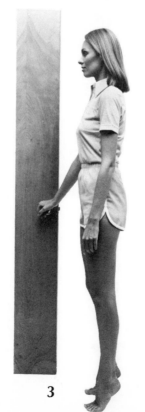

2

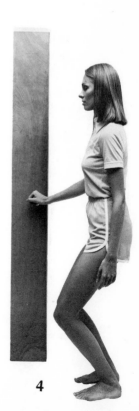

4

## 2.

### The Foot-Roll Prance

Stand with your feet parallel, 2 to 3 inches apart. Roll up onto the ball of one foot, bending your knee. Continue to roll up to a pointed position, with the tips of your toes a few inches above the ground. Try rolling through your foot a few times at a slow tempo. Then do it as a springing action, pushing the floor away. Do four or five of these movements on each of your feet, alternating them, if you like.

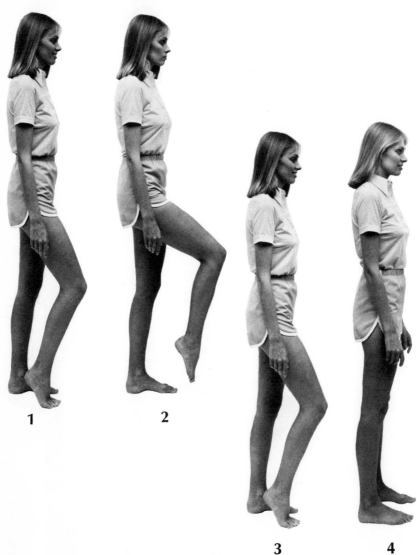

1                    2

3                    4

Go back to the slow tempo, raising your thigh higher and higher until it's at a 90-degree angle with your body. This should be done very quietly, as if you were tip-toeing. When you gently replace your foot on the floor, don't lock your knee. Do twenty or thirty of these.

This exercise warms up the muscles of the feet and legs. In addition, it trains the coordination of the feet for running and jumping.

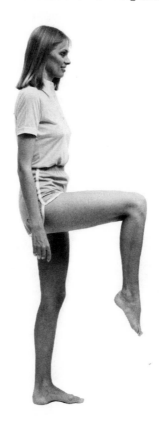

## 3.

## The Squat

Stand facing something you can hold onto, a doorknob for example. Now, place your feet parallel about 18 inches apart. Stand 6 to 8 inches away from the door, take hold of the doorknob, and lean back slightly. Keep your back upright and your heels on the floor, and squat down all the way. Make sure that your knees don't turn in. Keep them directly over your feet. Exhale as you squat, and remain there for a second. Inhale as you're coming back up. Do this ten or fifteen times.

As you go down, allow your head to come slightly forward so that you are looking at the floor between you and the door. This will prevent you from compressing the back of your neck. If you have strong thighs and are sufficiently flexible in the hip joint, you can do this exercise without holding onto anything. However, for warming-up purposes, it is slightly preferable to hold onto something. Try to hold the doorknob or another object as gently as possible. Use it only for balance, not to support your weight.

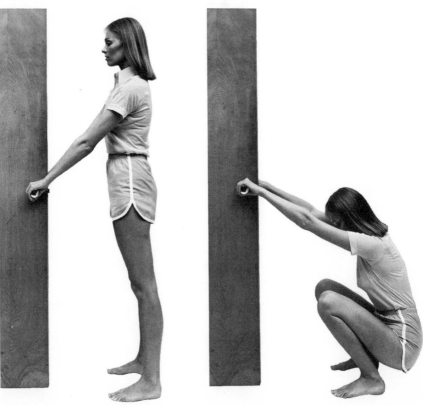

4.

## The Backward Brush

Standing parallel, place one foot about 6 to 8 inches in front of the other and drag your foot backward, exerting moderate pressure with the sole of your foot on the floor. This movement resembles someone propelling a scooter, or a feisty dog kicking up dirt with his back paws, or a bull preparing for the charge. As you drag your foot back and into the air, it should create a brushing sound. Keep it on the floor as long as possible. Your body will naturally lean forward a little. Alternate right and left legs ten or fifteen times.

This exercise warms up the calf, back thigh, and lower-back muscles.

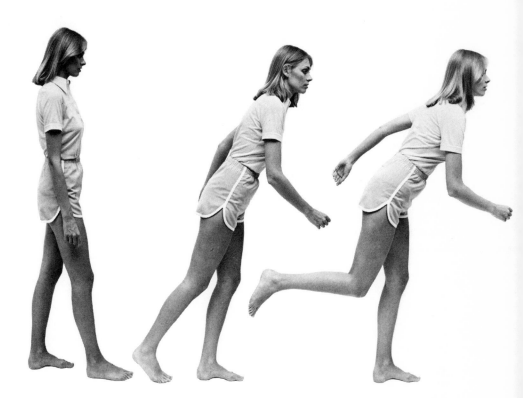

5.

## The Heel Spring

Stand with your feet parallel, 2 or 3 inches apart. To begin, bend your knees and make sure that your heels remain on the ground before you jump. Then spring into the air so that your toes are an inch off the floor. Roll through the foot both going up and coming down, as you did with the Foot Roll Prance.

It's absolutely essential that you push off from your whole foot (heel on the floor) rather than just from the balls of your feet. Upon landing, it's crucial that you roll through your feet and let your heels sink into the floor. Don't let the heels bounce up when you land. Jumping in sports and exercise activities without properly following these two central rules causes many injuries to the foot and lower leg. Your jump and especially your landing should be fairly quiet. If your heel slams into the floor and there is a loud smashing noise, something is wrong. Also, in order to protect your knees and ankles, make sure that your knees bend directly over your feet. (Proper alignment of the knee and ankle are more completely explained in the chapter on alignment, page 189.)

Do ten to fifteen Heel Springs, rest for a moment, and then try it again. As you become stronger, you can increase the number of sets to elevate your heart rate.

The Heel Spring warms up the muscles of your legs, hips, and back. You also begin to warm up your respiratory and cardiovascular systems. Most important, you start to coordinate many muscles and joints in a unified fashion, and all of your muscles begin to be integrated for your sports activity.

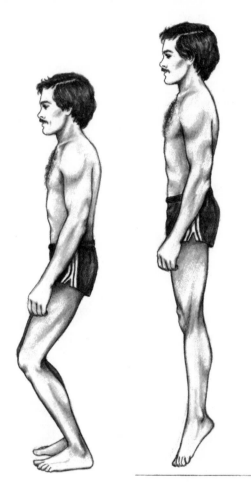

## 6.

### The Knee Swingout

Stand with your feet parallel and 2 to 3 inches apart, with hands on hips. Lift your knee in an arc from front to side so that your thigh ends up perpendicular to your trunk. Now, retracing your original arc, return your leg to the standing position. If balancing is difficult, hold onto something. Do eight to ten lifts with each leg, and repeat, if you'd like to.

The Knee Swingout warms up all the muscles of the front thigh, the inner thigh, and the hip. This exercise also enhances the lubrication of the hip joint.

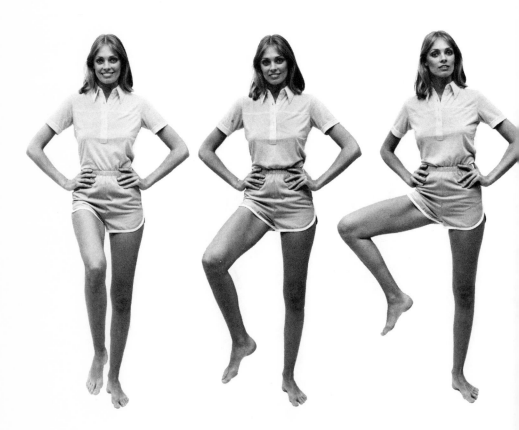

# 7.

## Running in Place with a Spring

Try to read these directions through as if you have no idea of how to run in place.

As you begin to run in place, it's best to make relatively small movements. Also, occasionally glance down to make sure that your feet are parallel and that your knees are not turned in. The knees should be facing straight ahead. On each run, roll through the foot, as in the Heel Springs. If you can move through the foot without crashing down, you will diminish the shock to your body by 80 percent. Keep your mouth slightly open, and breathe through it and your nose simultaneously.

About every fifteenth run, begin to spring up as if you're jumping over something with each step. The jumps should be slight, and moderately paced. Don't do them like you're leaping over hurdles. Over the course of the exercise, lift your feet higher and higher.

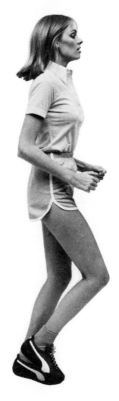

Alternate approximately fifteen to twenty relaxed jogs with about five or six springing light runs. The latter should be done at a slightly slower pace. Do two or three sets with small steps, and then two or three sets with the legs lifted higher. This entire exercise should take from thirty seconds to a maximum of two or three minutes.

Running in Place culminates the sequence of lower-body warm-up exercises. It increases the heart and respiratory rates, and works the muscles of the entire body in a coordinated fashion. If your physical activities use principally the lower part of the body, you should now be ready to go. Have fun.

## THE UPPER-BODY WARM-UP

# 1.

## Arm Circles

Stand with your left foot about 12 inches in front of your right, and swing the right arm in a circle as if you were winding up to pitch a softball. Keep the elbow fairly straight but not locked. Gradually increase your speed. Circle fifteen or twenty times, then reverse your leg position and swing the other arm. Now return to your original position and swing your right arm in the other direction. Then repeat on the other side. Rest for a moment in between each set.

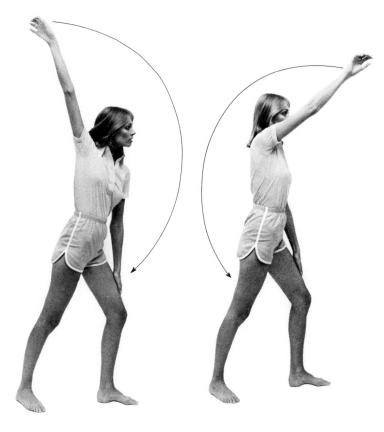

## 2.

### Double Arm Circles

Stand with your feet parallel, about 2 feet apart. Bend your knees slightly and lean forward about 6 inches. Alternating arms, circle them in the overhand-pitch direction. As you do this one, your arms move inward as they circle to the front so that your hands move past your face one after the other. Let the movement be continuous as if you were a windmill, circling about fifteen or twenty times. Don't forget to breathe and relax your neck.

Both Arm-Circle exercises warm up the muscles of the chest, upper arm, and shoulders, and they flood the muscles of the arms and hands with extra blood, due to centrifugal force. They loosen tension in the shoulder muscles and increase the secretion of fluid within the shoulder joints.

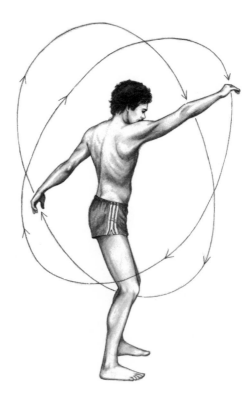

## 3.

## The Waist Twist

Skip this one if you tend to get lower-back pain. Stand with your feet parallel and about 18 inches apart. Bring your arms out to the side and swing them as you twist your upper body to the right as far as it will go, turning your head as well. Bend your knees slightly as you complete the twist. Your arms should be relaxed enough to swing freely and wrap around your body. At the end of each twist, bend both arms at the elbow so that the forearms gently touch your body.

When you've gone as far as you can to the right, swing your body to the left. Keep a brisk pace, with your body moving first and your arms following. Gradually increase the speed of the twist and don't move your feet. Do this exercise ten to twenty times.

This exercise warms up and loosens the muscles of the waist, lower back, and shoulders.

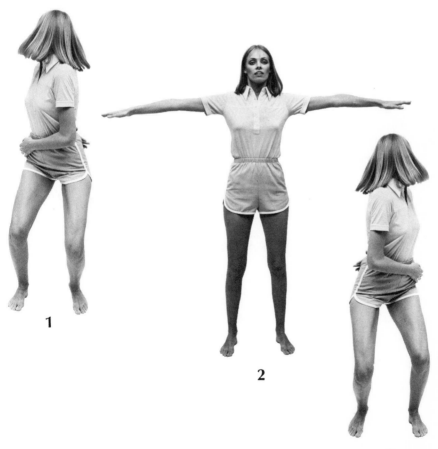

1

2

3

4.

## The Chest Stretch

Stand with your feet together and parallel, your weight over the balls of your feet. Extend your hands in front of your chest with the fingertips gently touching. Open the arms quickly to the sides, moving them slightly up and back beyond the shoulders until you reach your extreme stretch. Release slightly for an instant and reach quickly back again. As you open your arms, exhale through your mouth and raise your heels about an inch off the ground. Return to the starting position, inhaling as you bring your fingertips together. Rest for a moment and repeat. Do this eight or ten times.

The Chest Stretch warms up the muscles of the chest, shoulders, and upper back and increases the flexibility of the pectoral muscles.

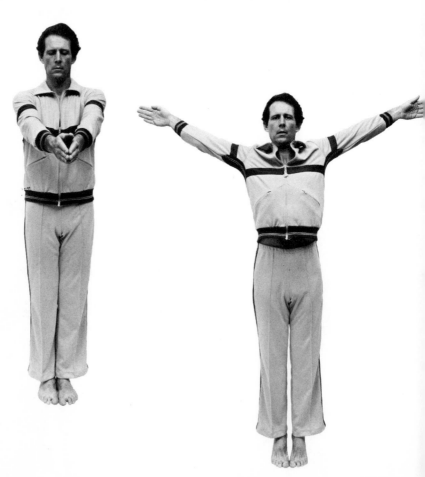

## 5.

### Hand Flexion

Throughout this exercise, keep your hand and fingers completely straight and your fingers together. Bend only at the wrist. Hold your arm in front of you, either bent at the elbow or straight, and flex your hand up to the extreme as if you were a traffic cop saying Stop. Move only the hand, not the arm. Extend it out, then down as far as it will go in the opposite direction. Repeat about eight or ten times. Then, try the other hand. Return to the first hand and begin the second phase with it up and back as far as it can go. Now, release it about a half-inch and flex it again in a continuous pulsating action, five or six times. Now bend the hand into the extreme down position and repeat again. Now try the other hand.

This exercise warms up the muscles of the forearm and the wrist joint.

## 6.

## The Back Curl Reach

Stand with your feet parallel, about 12 inches apart. Simultaneously bend your knees, exhale through your mouth, round your back, and extend your arms forward so that they are parallel to the floor. Allow your head to bend forward so you are looking between your knees. Exhale audibly on the curl and move moderately fast. Now simultaneously inhale, roll up through your back, and let your arms come gently to your sides to return to the starting position. Do this returning action slowly. Repeat this exercise eight or ten times.

This exercise warms up the body generally, with an emphasis on the back.

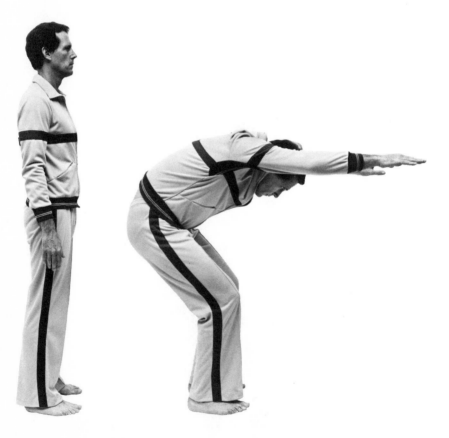

## THE UPPER-LOWER COMBINATION WARM-UP

The upper-lower combination warm-up is a selected series of the previous exercises designed to prepare you for those activities which use the upper and lower parts of the body with equal demand. Do this series after the general body warm-up.

1.   ARM CIRCLES, page 87
2.   DOUBLE ARM CIRCLES, page 88
3.   THE WAIST TWIST, page 89
4.   HAND FLEXION, page 91
5.   THE BACK CURL REACH, page 92
6.   THE KNEE BEND AND RAISE, page 76
7.   THE FOOT-ROLL PRANCE (small and high), page 78
8.   THE BACKWARD BRUSH, page 81
9.   RUNNING IN PLACE WITH A SPRING (small and big), page 85

## THE DANCE WARM-UP

This special series of warm-ups can be done before any kind of dance class or before an exercise or yoga class. Do the series after the general body warm-up.

1.   ARM CIRCLES, page 87
2.   THE WAIST TWIST, page 89
3.   THE CHEST STRETCH, page 90
4.   THE BACK CURL REACH, page 92
5.   THE KNEE BEND AND RAISE, page 76
6.   THE FOOT-ROLL PRANCE (small and high), page 78
7.   THE SQUAT, page 80
8.   THE BACKWARD BRUSH, page 81
9.   THE KNEE SWINGOUT, page 84

## SUMMARY OF WARM-UP PROGRAMS

**THE GENERAL WARM-UP**

1. Breathing
2. Toe Flexion
3. Ankle Circles
4. Ankle Flexion
5. Foot-Shaking
6A. The Knee-to-Chest
6B. The Knee-to-Chest, with a Foot Throw
6C. Chest, Extend, Chest, Replace
7. The Pelvic Tilt and Lift
8. Chest, Extend, Lift, Replace
9. Chest, Circle Out, Extend, Replace
10. The Lower-Back Twist
11. The Bicycle
12. The Sky Reach
13. The Side Reach
14. Shoulder Rolls
15. The Shoulder Drop
16. Hand-Shaking
17. The Head Compass

**THE LOWER-BODY WARM-UP**

1. The Knee Bend and Raise
2. The Foot-Roll Prance
3. The Squat
4. The Backward Brush
5. The Heel Spring
6. The Knee Swingout
7. Running in Place with a Spring

**THE UPPER-BODY WARM-UP**

1. Arm Circles
2. Double Arm Circles
3. The Waist Twist
4. The Chest Stretch
5. Hand Flexion
6. The Back Curl Reach

**THE UPPER-LOWER COMBINATION WARM-UP**

1. Arm Circles
2. Double Arm Circles
3. The Waist Twist
4. Hand Flexion
5. The Back Curl Reach
6. The Knee Bend and Raise
7. The Foot-Roll Prance
8. The Backward Brush
9. Running in Place with a Spring

**THE DANCE WARM-UP**

1. Arm Circles
2. The Waist Twist
3. The Chest Stretch
4. The Back Curl Reach
5. The Knee Bend and Raise
6. The Foot-Roll Prance
7. The Squat
8. The Backward Brush
9. The Knee Swingout

# 5

# YOUR OWN
# FITNESS PROFILE

Warming up before sports and exercise is the best way to avoid pain and injury. Sometimes, however, additional help is needed, especially when certain areas of your body are tight, out of alignment, or prone to frequent injury. In this chapter, I have provided a fitness test to help you determine your vulnerable areas. Once you know where you need some extra work, you can strengthen and improve your weak spots with the specific information in Chapters 6 through 10.

General fitness is the sum total of many aspects. It includes flexibility, good alignment, cardiovascular fitness, strength, and a minimum of muscular tension. The following series of tests are designed to show you: (1) exactly where in your body you hold destructive tension; (2) where your muscles are stretched and flexible* and where they're not; (3) where your postural alignment is on or off; (4) and your degree of vulnerability to injury in the various segments of your body. Each part of the body will be tested separately where possible. These four areas will be covered, followed by an analysis of the test results in each category and recommendations for change. All four influence the quality of your performance and your susceptibility to injury in very important ways.

*The term *flexible* is customarily used to refer to joint mobility. In this book, however, *flexible* has been used to describe muscle pliancy and suppleness, except where indicated.

**95**

The tests in this section cover those areas which can be objectively determined. Strength and endurance are matters of individual need. Everyone needs a different amount of strength depending on the need of his or her life-style. It is my belief that strength can and should be maintained by your activities and does not need to be developed artificially in isolated exercise or weight-lifting programs for general body maintenance. Strength exercises in the context of this book are used primarily to help you in a new athletic or exercise program, or to return after an injury or a prolonged break.

I recommend that you have a complete medical checkup and an analysis of your cardiovascular fitness before embarking upon any vigorous exercise program.

In order to make the most productive use of this book, it is important that you take the tests and analyze the results. Don't try to get a good score by stretching the truth. Be as honest as you can and ask somebody's help if you don't know the answers to some questions— for instance, your posture is sometimes hard to see by yourself.

It is important to avoid exercises that may hurt you, and these tests will help you to find out what they are. Working the wrong way is a waste of time and energy and can lead to injury. You may think you have a problem with strength, but it might just be muscle tension holding you back. You may feel tense, but the real problem could be postural alignment. You may know your problem exactly, but be working on it backward, never understanding why you're not getting anywhere. If your body is not prepared, you may at best stretch ineffectively and accomplish nothing, and at worst injure yourself.

The exercises and recommendations made in each test analysis are detailed in the Tension-Relaxation, Stretching, Strength, and Alignment chapters that follow. Professional help is recommended for certain tension and postural alignment problems. A description of various therapeutic modalities I recommend for helping these particular problems can be found in the Appendix.

## THE FEET AND ANKLES

### Tension

1. Are your feet often cold? Yes _____ No _____
2. Do you ever get cramps in your feet? Yes _____ No _____
3. Do they often hurt when you stand for several hours at a time? Yes _____ No _____
4. Are your feet extremely ticklish? Yes _____ No _____

If you answered yes to any of the above questions, there is probably considerable tension in your feet. To correct foot tension, refer to the section on the legs and feet (page 129) in Chapter 6.

### Joint Flexibility

1. Can you stand on the extreme outsides of your feet easily with your knees slightly bent? Yes _____ No _____
2. Are your ankles wobbly or do you easily fall over on them when you lose your footing? Yes _____ No _____
3. Do you have a high instep? Yes _____ No _____

If you answered yes to at least two questions here, the joints of your foot and ankle tend to be a little too flexible. To increase stability you should build extra strength in your feet and lower legs, using the exercises described on page 163 in Chapter 8.

### Alignment

1. Hold onto something for balance. With your feet parallel and two inches apart, rise up on the balls of your feet. Do your ankles tend either to roll out toward the small toes or in toward the big toes? Yes _____ No _____
2. Do you have flat feet or fallen arches? (If they're flat or fallen, while you stand you won't be able to slide your finger in an inch under your arch.) Yes _____ No _____
3. Do you walk with your feet turned out? Yes _____ No _____

If you answered yes to at least two questions in this section, your movement is affected by poor foot and ankle alignment. This means that your ankle joint is constantly under considerable stress, especially when you walk or run. See the section on the ankle (page 189) in Chapter 9 for corrective exercises.

## Vulnerability

1. Do you ever get pain or strain in the ankle, heel, or arch of the foot? Yes ＿＿ No ＿＿
2. Do your feet fall asleep or do you feel "pins and needles" in them fairly often? Yes ＿＿ No ＿＿
3. Have you ever had a foot injury; pain in the ankle, heel, arch; strains, or the like? Yes ＿＿ No ＿＿
4. Do you regularly experience small nagging pains in your feet during normal activity or while exercising? Yes ＿＿ No ＿＿

If you answered yes here, it means that your feet and ankles are already quite vulnerable to injury. Be especially careful to warm up this area before exercising. Spend extra time on it. See the section on lower-body warm-up, and concentrate on the foot and ankle strengthening series (page 163) in Chapter 8.

## THE LOWER LEGS AND KNEES

### Tension

1. Do your lower legs often get tired when standing?
   Yes ＿＿ No ＿＿
2. Do you experience cramps in your calves with any regularity?
   Yes ＿＿ No ＿＿
3. Do you trip over things a lot? Yes ＿＿ No ＿＿
4. Sit in a chair and cross your legs so that the ankle of your left foot is resting on top of your right thigh just above the knee. Now grip your lower leg so that the tips of your thumbs press into the center of your calf. Squeeze your leg so that your thumb tips press quite firmly into the calf. Does that hurt? (Try the other leg.)
   Yes ＿＿ No ＿＿
5. Remaining in approximately the same position, press the tips of all your fingers into the center of your shin muscles. Does that hurt? Yes ＿＿ No ＿＿

If you answered yes to at least two questions, it means that your lower leg is tense. The more questions you answered yes to, the more tension there probably is in this area. Calf and shin tension generally go together, but the places where you feel the most discomfort indicate which section is tighter. Unless the chronic tension in this area is reduced, you endanger the safety of both the knee and the ankle. Elevating the legs and taking warm baths (as described on pages 37 and 35) are a must every day for people with lower-leg tension. In addition, see the relaxation exercises for the legs (page 129) in the tension-relaxation chapter. You will be particularly prone to injury if you do any running without a thorough warm-up. Calf tension is particularly stubborn and hard to get rid of without some professional assistance, so see the Appendix if your problem persists.

## Muscle and Joint Flexibility

1. Stand disrobed from the waist down so you can see your legs and feet. Look down and place your feet absolutely parallel about two inches apart. Now bend your knees as far as you can with your heels remaining on the ground and your back upright. Drop your head and look down. Is it difficult for you to move your knees apart so that you can see all five toes on each foot? Yes _____ No _____

2. While sitting, straighten your leg and flex your foot as far as you can. Does it hurt your calf if you hold this position for two or three seconds? Yes _____ No _____

3. Do you have hyperextended knees? (This means that when you straighten your knee it locks and looks as if it is bowed slightly backward.) Yes _____ No _____

If you have answered yes to any question here, your calves are not very stretched. This may also indicate tension in the calf. Work on lower-leg stretching (page 141), detailed in Chapter 7.

## Alignment

1. Do you walk with your feet completely parallel? Yes _____ No _____

2. Stand in the bent-knee position described in Question 1 under Flexibility, above. Can you see your two or two and a half toes on

the inside of your feet without moving your knees, as shown in the accompanying diagram? Yes _____ No _____

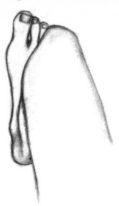

If you answered no to either of these questions, you have poor knee-foot alignment. This means that during physical activity, including walking, stress is placed on the knee joint, especially on the inside of the knee. If you try standing with your feet quite turned out and then bend your knees in a forward direction as far as you can, holding this position for a few moments, you will begin to feel stress on the inner knee in addition to the ankle. The more force going through your leg when it is misaligned, the more the knee is stressed, increasing the danger progressively from walking to running to jumping. Correction of knee and lower-leg alignment is crucial to safe movement habits, especially in athletics and dance. As a result of poor alignment one often develops tension and muscular imbalance. Take extra time in concentrating on the alignment chapter. If you have hyperextended knees, try to get professional help to correct this problem. This will help to prevent injuries to the knee and tension buildup in the lower leg.

## Vulnerability

1. Have you had shin splints or severe pain in the front lower leg more than once in your life? Yes _____ No _____
2. Have you ever suffered severe pain or spasm in the calf that lasted for more than a day? Yes _____ No _____
3. Do your calves or shins feel sore frequently after exercising? Yes _____ No _____

4. Have you ever sustained a knee injury or had frequent recurring pain in the knee? Yes _____ No _____
5. Have you ever injured or strained your Achilles tendon (the cordlike structure that attaches the calf muscle to the back of the heel)? Yes _____ No _____

If you answered yes here, to any question, you have already pushed your lower legs beyond their limit at some time. This leaves you more vulnerable to other injuries of the knee, lower leg, and ankle. If you have had knee problems, stay away from the lotus position in yoga. It places unnatural stress on the knee joint. Concentrate on your alignment or tension problems. Always warm up before exertion, and make some of the body-care techniques in Chapter 2 part of your daily routine.

## THE THIGHS

### Tension

1. If someone were to forcefully grip and squeeze your thigh just above the front of your knee, would that hurt, tickle, or make you jump? (If you don't know, have someone try it).
   Yes _____ No _____
2. Do your thighs frequently feel sore in the front or back after vigorous exercise or stretching? Yes _____ No _____
3. Do you ever get cramps in the thigh? Yes _____ No _____
4. Do your thigh muscles bulge out sharply from the leg, especially just above the knees? Yes _____ No _____
5. Sit down and completely relax your leg. Squeeze your thigh muscles with your hand, front and back. Do they feel hard and taut? Yes _____ No _____

If you answered yes to any of these, you have thigh tension. If tension is present on the front of the thigh, it is generally also on the back thigh, although one will probably be dominant. This of course will be indicated by where you feel discomfort. Work to eliminate the tension in your thighs by using the techniques described on page 129. Regular Water Kicking is probably the best therapy.

## Flexibility

1. If you grasp the top of your foot and pull it up behind you while standing, can you touch your heel to your buttocks?
Yes ____ No ____
2. While sitting in a chair, grasp the front of one ankle with your knee slightly bent. Can you touch your knee to your forehead without much discomfort or difficulty? Yes ____ No ____
3. While lying on your back, is it easy for you to pull your knee to your chest? Yes ____ No ____
4. Sit on the floor with your legs extended in front of you. With your legs relaxed but fairly straight, can you take hold of your ankles easily, without much discomfort in the backs of the thighs?
Yes ____ No ____
5. While sitting on the floor with your legs spread apart, can you easily open them more than ninety degrees? Yes ____ No ____

If you answered no to any here, your thighs could use more stretch and muscle flexibility. Question 1 is for flexibility in the front thigh. This is not as crucial as hamstring flexibility, pinpointed in Questions 2 to 4, which is required for many athletics and exercise activities. Question 5 refers to inner-thigh flexibility, especially required in such activities as dance or karate. Tight hamstrings make you very prone to injury in the knees and lower back as well as the thighs, so you should try to obtain the maximum flexibility in these muscles. The manner in which you stretch them is crucial. Avoid hamstring stretches that are done in a standing position or that involve forcing or bouncing. For safe hamstring and thigh stretches, to improve flexibility, see those described in the stretch chapter (page 144). Developing flexible hamstrings is the best way to avoid pulled hamstrings.

## Vulnerability

1. Have you ever had a pulled hamstring or inner-thigh muscle that gave you trouble for more than a day or two? Yes ____ No ____
2. Did you ever have pain that lasted more than a day or so in the upper inner thigh near the groin, or at the front of the hip joint (at the very top of your leg), especially while walking?
Yes ____ No ____
3. Did you ever have a severe accident and break your thigh bone (the femur)? Yes ____ No ____

4.  Have you ever had a thigh operation? Do you have a steel pin in your thigh or hip joint? Yes _____ No _____

If you answered yes to any question here, your knee, thigh, hip, and lower-back areas will be more vulnerable to injury. Previous tears in muscles often heal poorly and maintain inherent weaknesses, especially if there is a lot of scar tissue. If you have been injured before and wish to continue being very active, work on the tension in your thighs and make thigh, calf, and lower-back stretching (Chapter 7) a regular part of your exercise regime, *at the end of your physical activity.*

## THE LOWER BACK, PELVIS, AND ABDOMEN

### Tension

1.  Stand up and dig your thumb into your buttock muscles. Do they feel tough or hard, or does it hurt? Yes _____ No _____
2.  Do you usually keep your buttock muscles contracted while standing? Yes _____ No _____
3.  Stand with your feet parallel and two inches apart. Bend your knees slightly and place one hand on your abdomen and one on your buttocks. Now try to make the buttocks and abdomen completely soft and loose. While remaining upright, try to swing your pelvis forward and back. Don't lean with your body. Does moving your pelvis in this way cause you to tighten your abdomen or buttock muscles? Use your fingers to check.
    Yes _____ No _____
4.  Do you generally try to hold your stomach in while you are standing up? Yes _____ No _____
5.  Do you get cramps in your abdominal area—whether menstrual or otherwise—with any regularity? Yes _____ No _____
6.  Does your lower back ache or get stiff or tired very easily?
    Yes _____ No _____

Tense areas in the lower back, hips, and abdominal area often occur together. If you answered yes to any of these questions, there is a good deal of tension and stress placed on your lower back and pelvic region. Thus, you are vulnerable to lower-back and hip injuries and should pay special attention to pages 123–24 on tension-relaxation, and pages

198–201 on alignment. Swimming and kicking in the water on your back are probably the best exercises for you. Nightly warm baths are also helpful. Special care should always be taken when you lift things—bend at the knees and not at the waist. Forceful stretching can also be very dangerous.

## Flexibility

1. While sitting, does twisting your shoulders to face the wall squarely to the right of you and then to the left of you cause any discomfort? Yes ـــــ No ـــــ
2. In a standing position, can you pull your knee up to touch your chest? Yes ـــــ No ـــــ
3. Standing with your feet parallel and together, can you bend to the left and touch the outside of your left knee with your left hand without discomfort in the right lower back and waist? Try it on the other side also. Yes ـــــ No ـــــ

When there is limited flexibility in the lower back, it is frequently due to tension and not to lack of stretch. If you answered no to any of the above questions, you have limited flexibility in the lower back. If turning the upper body while in a stationary position is difficult, you will be particularly prone to lower-back injury, especially in hitting a ball with a bat or in tennis. Gently work on flexibility here by paying special attention to the Side Reach (page 71), the standing lower-back Waist Twist (page 89), the floor Lower-Back Twist (page 66), and the Pelvic Tilt and Lift (page 58).

## Alignment

1. Stand sideways in front of a mirror with your feet parallel and two or three inches apart. Do you have a swayback? Does your abdomen drop forward? Do your buttocks protrude in the back and is there an accentuated curve in the small of your back? (This posture is also referred to as lordosis, hyperextension of the back, or a swayback). Yes ـــــ No ـــــ
2. Standing sideways in front of a mirror with your feet parallel and two to three inches apart, is your lower back completely flat with no curve? Does the pelvis look tucked under, flattening the buttocks? Yes ـــــ No ـــــ
3. When standing, do you usually sit into one hip?
   Yes ـــــ No ـ――

If you answered yes to Question 1 and you have some lordosis, there is constant stress on the lower-back vertebrae and discs. This posture perpetuates tension in the lower-back muscles. If you sit into one hip when you stand, as in Question 3, you constantly create tension. If you answered yes to Question 2 and your lower back is flat with the pelvis slung forward, you probably carry your weight in your thighs, resulting in extra tension or bulk there. You may also compensate for this by collapsing your chest and center back. Correction of these alignment problems is important to assure safety during exercise, and is covered in the lower-back and pelvic section (page 198) of the alignment chapter.

## Vulnerability

1. Have you ever had a lower-back or hip injury with pain or spasm? Yes _____ No _____
2. Have you ever had pain which radiated through your hip, or down your leg? Yes _____ No _____
3. Do you get little lower-back aches and pains, either after a long day or when you wake up in the morning? Yes _____ No _____
4. Have you ever had a lower-back or hip operation? Yes _____ No _____
5. Have you ever had ulcerative disorders in your stomach or intestines? Yes _____ No _____

If you answered yes to any of these questions, your lower-back region has an increased susceptibility to injury. Serious injuries to the lower back usually follow minor problems that often recur over a period of years. The causes are most often tension and alignment. Warming up before exercising is crucial for people with lower-back difficulties. If you have trouble with any of the warm-up exercises such as the Lower-Back Twist and the Standing Waist Twist, either eliminate them or put them at the end of your warm-up. If you have to strain, don't do it. Spend extra time warming up your lower back, especially concentrating on the Chest, Extend, Chest, Replace; the Pelvic Tilt and Lift; the Chest, Extend, Lift, Replace; and the Chest, Circle Out, Extend, Replace general warm-up exercises (pages 57–62). Avoid exercises which place abnormal stress and tension on the lower back, such as double leg lifts, or the cobra in yoga.

## THE CHEST AND CENTER BACK

### Tension

1. Do you have difficulty while breathing, or feel constriction in your chest? (This is sometimes perceived as a tight band around the chest.) Yes _____ No _____
2. Do you get winded easily while exercising? Yes _____ No _____
3. Do you frequently get a stitch in your side during vigorous activity? Yes _____ No _____
4. Do you spend many hours a day in a bent-over position typing, writing, or leaning over a work table? Yes _____ No _____
5. Take your left hand and firmly squeeze your right pectoral muscle between your thumb and forefingers. This is located just in front of the underarm. Does that hurt? Yes _____ No _____
6. Do you ever have pain between the shoulder blades?
   Yes _____ No _____

If you answered yes to any of these questions, there is some excess tension in your chest and center-back area. We often think of our ribs as being only in the front of our bodies, but our rib cage encases the upper torso and attaches to the spine in the back. When there is breathing restriction due to tension, center- or upper-back problems often follow. Tension often manifests itself circularly around the body. If a breathing restriction is extreme, it often indicates deeply rooted emotional problems. But if it is somewhat minor, tension-release and relaxation exercises are often very helpful. For those with minor problems in the middle and upper back, the Large-Ball Chest Release on page 122 is often extremely helpful. It must be done daily. I also suggest that the Small-Ball Techniques (page 125) and the upper-body warm-ups (pages 87–92) be done daily, even twice a day. They take four or five minutes and can be done without the general warm-up preceding them.

### Flexibility

Take a thick, bath-sized towel and keep folding it until it is tightly packed into approximately a six-inch square at least four inches in height. Place the folded towel over your spine at your center back. Now lie down on your back on the floor. With the towel still under you, open your arms to the side and lie there for about ten seconds. Does it hurt or feel uncomfortable in your chest or center back? Yes _____ No _____

The concept of muscle and joint flexibility is not easily applied to the chest and center back. Although there is some flexibility, the ribs are fixed into the spine and leave this segment of the body with limited range of movement. Lack of flexibility usually indicates tension rather than unstretched muscles, and it can be improved with the use of the Large-Ball Chest Release (page 122).

## Alignment

1. Do you generally stand slouched over, exaggerating your center-back curve? This usually occurs with a slightly collapsed chest and round-shoulderedness. Look in the mirror or ask a friend. Yes _____ No _____
2. Do you try to stand with your chest held up and your stomach pulled in? Yes _____ No _____
3. Stand up and take your shirt or blouse off and look at your lower ribs. Do they stick out a little bit? Yes _____ No _____

If you answered yes to Question 1, it generally indicates poor alignment through habit. Poor center-back and chest alignment is a major factor in lower-back pain. See the section on chest alignment (page 202) for corrective exercises. Questions 2 and 3, a chronically high-held chest and protruding ribs, indicate tension. Try the Large-Ball Chest Release (page 122) and the Small-Ball Techniques for the upper and center back (pages 125–26).

## THE SHOULDERS

### Tension

1. Do you notice a stiffness or tightness in your shoulders fairly often? Yes _____ No _____
2. Are your arms often asleep when you wake up? Yes _____ No _____
3. Forcefully squeeze the top of your left shoulder (the muscle

between the base of your neck and the tip of your shoulder) with your right hand. Then do your right shoulder. Does that hurt? Yes _____ No _____

4.  Do you ever notice that you raise your shoulders up when you are doing simple activities such as writing, lifting things, or concentrating intently? Yes _____ No _____

If you answered yes to any question here, you have tension in your shoulders and upper-back area, and you are prone to pains and injuries in the shoulder joints, such as torn tendons, bursitis, and arthritis. Doing shoulder-relaxation exercises (page 120) several times throughout the day is often helpful, and frequent use of the upper-body warmup exercises daily to increase blood circulation and awareness in the shoulders is also good.

## Flexibility

1.  Lie prone on the floor and place one hand in the middle of your lower back. Now relax. Does your elbow touch the floor? Yes _____ No _____
2.  Put your right hand behind you as if you were in a hammer lock. Now put your left hand over your left shoulder. Can you reach and touch the fingers of your right and left hands? Yes _____ No _____

If you answered no to either of these questions, you probably have some loss of flexibility in the shoulder. Since the shoulder is attached to the body primarily by muscles, inflexibility and limitation of movement range here are most often caused by excess muscle tension, so follow the procedures described under shoulder tension, above.

## Alignment

1.  Are you round-shouldered? Yes _____ No _____
2.  Look in the mirror carefully. Is one shoulder higher than the other? Yes _____ No _____
3.  Do you try to pull your shoulders back when you are standing? Yes _____ No _____

If you answered yes to any of the questions in this section, your shoulder girdle does not hang squarely on your body and is out of alignment. The slouched shoulder is often related to the collapsed chest (page 202), and should be handled in the same manner.

## Vulnerability

1. Have you ever had a shoulder injury or chronic shoulder pain? Yes _____ No _____
2. Do you feel occasional pain in your shoulder, shoulder joint, or upper-back area at least once a week? Yes _____ No _____
3. Have you ever dislocated your shoulder? Yes _____ No _____

If you already feel pain, or have ever injured your shoulder, you are more vulnerable to injury. Weakened ligaments are more easily strained again. If you are prone to pain here, always spend extra time on your upper-body warm-up before moving into more vigorous activity, and work on reducing your shoulder tension (page 120) or alignment (page 207) problems. This is the best protection you can have.

## THE ARMS AND HANDS

### Tension

1. Do your arms get tired very easily? Yes _____ No _____
2. Do they often suddenly feel weak? Yes _____ No _____
3. Do your hands get cold easily? Yes _____ No _____
4. Take the thumb and forefingers of the right hand and squeeze the triceps muscle, on the underside of the upper arm, fairly forcefully. Does that hurt? Yes _____ No _____
5. Do you fidget with your hands a lot—tapping them and playing with objects? Yes _____ No _____

If you answered yes to two or more, you have some excess tension. Tension in the arms and hands is usually related to the amount of tension in the shoulders, which blocks circulation to the arms and results in further tension buildup. In order to relax the arms and hands, you should concentrate on your shoulder tension. Do the upper-body warm-up frequently, and the Towel-Twisting and the Hand-Shaking exercises (pages 121–22) and even the Wrist Stretch and the Palm Press (pages 156–57) every day.

## Vulnerability

1. Have you ever broken or dislocated any of your fingers or broken your arm? Have you ever broken any bones in your wrist? Yes_____ No_____
2. Have you ever suffered from pains in your arms or hands? Yes _____ No _____
3. Do your hands tend to cramp up on you? Yes _____ No _____
4. Do you tend to cut or bruise your hands or bang them into things? Yes _____ No _____

Loss of feeling or sensitivity in the arms and hands often leads to other kinds of injury because your arms and hands protect your face during a sudden fall. Loss of sensitivity often results from tension which blocks blood circulation and disc injuries in the neck which impede nerve impulses. If you have had difficulties in this area already, you should be extremely careful if you play contact sports. One thing to remember if you have hurt your wrist before is not to bend it to the extreme during an exertive activity. Once it has been strained, it is usually very prone to reinjury. Always make a special effort to warm up your hands during the upper-body warm-ups. And do the strengthening exercises (page 182) regularly.

## THE NECK

### Tension

1. Do you get headaches once a month or more? Yes _____ No _____
2. Do you grind your teeth? Yes _____ No _____
3. Grasp the back of your neck and squeeze it fairly forcefully. Does it hurt or feel hard? Yes _____ No _____
4. Do you crack your neck all the time? Yes _____ No _____
5. Does your neck generally feel tight and stiff? Yes _____ No _____

If you answered yes to any of these questions, your neck is somewhat tense and thus you have a precondition for stiff necks, neck spasms, and intense pain which may radiate from the neck into the shoulder or hand. Be careful of any exercises that place all or most of your weight on your neck vertebrae, such as shoulder stands and head stands. Neck circling exercises should also be avoided because the circling movement from side to back and then back to the side can be dangerous. Neck tension is often the forerunner of teeth grinding, or bruxism. To relieve chronic neck tension, try the exercises described on pages 116–19, but therapeutic help (see Appendix) is often required. A device I developed called the Neck Relaxer is also extremely helpful in reducing neck tension.

## Flexibility

1. Are you uncomfortable lying prone with your head to either side? Yes ____ No ____
2. Does your neck hurt when you look at the ceiling? Yes ____ No ____
3. While sitting upright, does touching your chin to your chest, keeping your mouth closed, cause any difficulty or discomfort? Yes ____ No ____

If you answered yes to Question 1, the rotational flexibility of your neck may be limited by tension or your bone structure. If you answered yes to Questions 2 or 3, your range of movement is probably limited by tension in your neck. In any case, the Neck Stretch (page 155) is recommended as are the suggestions for neck tension (page 116).

## Alignment

1. Stand sideways in front of a mirror and peek out of the corner of your eye. Is your head projected far forward? Yes ____ No ____
2. Now look straight in the mirror. Is your head slightly tilted to one side? Yes ____ No ____

If you answered yes and your head and neck are out of alignment, tension buildup in the neck is inevitable and susceptibility to injury in this area is greatly increased. Also, there are probably compensating spinal curves in the center and lower back that have been exaggerated. See pages 209–11 of the alignment chapter for recommended exercises.

### Vulnerability

1. Have you ever had a neck injury, or do you suffer pain in your neck with any frequency? Yes _____ No _____
2. Do you get stiff necks fairly frequently? Yes _____ No _____

If you answered yes here, you may have begun what is to be an accelerating chronic problem. Once you have had a neck injury there is greater effort required to make your neck safe from reinjury. You may have developed fear of being touched on the neck, making therapeutic help or even movement scary. You may have some actual damage. People often feel protective of their necks and develop more tension there. Work on your tension (page 116) and alignment (page 209) problems as suggested, and seek out professional help if you need it.

## CONCLUSION

Now that you have evaluated your test results, don't be discouraged. Comparing yourself to the ideal specimen can easily make you depressed. Just recognizing your problems and having clearly defined goals is half the solution. The test results provide you with concrete information to help you create a good corrective program.

Select the appropriate stretching, strengthening, alignment, relaxation, and warm-up exercises, but don't try to work on everything at once. Select one area of your body and work on it for about a month before proceeding to your next problem. Choose one problem and work on it until you understand it or until it begins to change. Then add something else.

If an area is both tense and inflexible, work on your tension first. It's difficult, if not impossible, to effectively stretch your muscles if they are very tense. I recommend taking the fitness profile test every six months to measure your progress.

The Muscular Therapy Institute offers a service for people who find it hard to organize their own fitness programs, and for those who need help with specific areas such as tension and alignment. The Institute analyzes your test results, and recommends an exercise program. It will also provide a list of individuals in your vicinity who are trained in areas that you may need help in.*

*For more information about this service, please write to the Muscular Therapy Institute, 910 West End Avenue, New York, N.Y. 10025.

# 6

# TENSION AND
# RELAXATION

At the moment before a stress-related injury, the body has already reached its capacity to absorb tension and will snap like a stick under pressure. The person who is both relaxed and strong stands the best chance of avoiding that injury.

Most people realize that excess tension prevents them from performing up to their potential. What is not known is that if you're chronically tense you stand a good chance of being injured while exercising. In fact, the probability of getting injured during exercise is ten times greater for people with chronic tension than for those with reduced tension levels. It's much more likely that you'll tear or sprain your muscles, ligaments, and tendons if your muscles are tense.

## WHAT IS MUSCULAR TENSION?

I often begin my self-care workshops and lectures on this subject by asking, "What would you be like without any tension?" I usually get such responses as: "I wouldn't be able to move," or "I couldn't get out of bed." A few students say, "I'd be like a vegetable." All of these answers are headed in the right direction but not taken far enough. Without any tension, you'd be dead.

*Muscular tension* is simply the contraction or moving together of muscle fibers. A muscle can only do one thing actively—contract. All the other things muscles do involve a letting go of tension. The ongoing contraction and release of muscle tension is necessary for life. Your heart is a muscle. Without the ability to contract and release, it would stop beating. If your diaphragm muscle stopped functioning, you'd stop breathing. The contraction and relaxation of muscle fiber is the source of all bodily movement, even for your eyelids. This cycle of tension and relaxation is the pulsation which pervades everything in life.

All of the muscles in your body that you can control are producing a constant and minute level of tension known as muscle tone. A muscle that is "in tone" isn't hard, mushy, or flabby; it's firm, but soft and pliant. When a muscle is not being used to move or support you, it should be capable of relaxing as much as possible. If a person has muscles that remain hard and constantly contracted, despite any attempts to release them, he is suffering from chronic excess tension, which seriously threatens his health and contributes to many "stress-related" diseases.

Excess tension is a constant and perpetual state that only fluctuates within a limited range. You don't stop being tense when you sit down, or even when you're asleep. If you suffer from chronic excess tension, you will be tense to various degrees all of the time.

## EFFECTS OF EXCESS TENSION

Excess tension holds you down; it prevents you from performing to your fullest in your favorite sport or exercise activity. Holding muscles contracted wastes a lot of energy. Even walking around in this state can be pretty tiring. Excess tension causes you to become prematurely fatigued in your game and it inhibits your body's movement. Tense muscles are inflexible and do not stretch easily, and this makes you more prone to injury.

Excess tension inhibits breathing and limits your oxygen intake. Chronically contracted chest and diaphragm muscles severely limit your wind and endurance. Each breath takes in less oxygen and expels less carbon dioxide.

Excess tension also slows down your reaction time, especially crucial in contact sports. It also interferes with physical sensations in general. Pressure from tense muscles often desensitizes small nerve endings throughout the body. Those whose reaction time is slower than they would like it to be are often suffering from excess tension. These individuals commonly incur major injuries. Excess tension often leads to the premature end of a career for athletes, and it also prevents them from reaching their fullest potential.

Excess tension blocks blood circulation. Blood is our lifeline, supplying oxygen and food to every cell in the body. It cleanses the body of carbon dioxide and other wastes. Good circulation lets you run that extra mile. When blood flow is poor, it takes longer to warm up and it's harder to stay warm. When your muscles become tense, they continually press on your blood vessels. This causes circulation to become less efficient. It's like trying to draw liquid through a pinched straw.

The danger of falling is a normal hazard of many sports. Relaxed muscles yield more easily to external force. Having muscles that are flexible enough to stretch to their full limit unimpeded by tension is good insurance against injury. You can never be completely safe, but with a relaxed body the percentages are in your favor. Out of a thousand skiers who suffer identical spills, only a small percentage rip cartilage in their knee joints. Some people can let their bodies go with the fall, while others resist and get injured. If your body is tense, your risk of injury is increased.

## EVERYBODY GETS TENSE

It's quite natural to get tense. It happens to everyone. You should be able to absorb and discharge small amounts of tension easily. Frequently, exercise is effective in ridding the body of superficial, day-to-day tension, which I call *current tension*.

*Chronic tension* is more deep seated, because it's been present for a long time. Generally, it's not affected by sports and exercise activities. Certain tension-release and relaxation exercises sometimes affect it positively, but people usually require professional help in eliminating their chronic tension.

Imagine that your body is a pail filled almost to the top with water. The water represents the amount of tension in your body. If the bucket is usually full, it means that there is a lot of chronic tension present. All you need is a little more water (tension) to make the bucket overflow (feel pain). If the bucket were one-eighth full of water, that would represent the amount of tension present for normal muscle tone. It's not the extra amount of tension that makes us overflow into pain, but the chronic tension that we have had for many years which gives us very little leeway for the normal tension buildup in our lives. If we begin with only the tension produced by normal muscle tone, we could double or triple our daily current tension without overflowing into a state of pain. It's natural for your body to move in and out of tension states, but it's not natural for these tension states to send you into pain.

What follows is a series of exercises designed to help you release excess tension in various parts of your body. Some of these exercises have been described in detail in other sections of the book and so will be referred to only by name. If you are interested in a more extensive selection of exercises for relaxation or tension-release exercises, see my book *Are You Tense?* (New York: Pantheon Books, 1977).

## THE NECK

## 1.

### The Block Technique

In order to do this exercise, you need a triangular block of wood approximately 3 inches high by 8 inches long. Each edge of the triangle should be constructed to exert different amounts of pressure; make one rounded, one semi-rounded, and one sharp.*

Please read the following instructions through completely before you begin this technique.

Lie on your back on the floor. Place the block on the floor, with the rounded edge facing up, directly under the back of your head. The rounded edge should be placed at your lower occipital line, which is where the base of the skull meets the neck (see diagram). As you lie on the block, try to relax the muscles of your neck. Don't tilt your head or try to hold your head up off the block.

If using the block is painful, place a washcloth over the edge of it to blunt the intensity of the edge. Later, when it's easier, discard the cloth.

Now, with your occiput on the rounded edge, roll your head very slowly, first to one side and then to the other. If you find a place that

*If you are unable to construct such a device yourself, you can purchase one, called a Neck Relaxer, for $17.00 from Relaxation Tools, Inc., P.O. Box 1045, New York, N.Y. 10025.

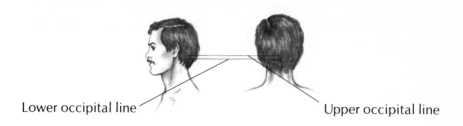

Lower occipital line                    Upper occipital line

hurts, leave your head there for ten to fifteen seconds, but never keep your head in one place longer than thirty seconds. Continue to roll your head, finding all the painful spots that you can. If it's too painful to stop at these points, a continual slow, rolling motion is often easier to tolerate at first. When all the discomfort on the lower occipital line ceases, repeat on the upper occipital line, a half-inch higher.

At first the block may slide or tip as you use it. If this occurs, *use one hand to stabilize it.* Placing the block on a rug may add further stability.

When the block no longer hurts on both occipital lines, try the semi-rounded edge. When this no longer causes pain on both lines, move to the sharpest edge, which exerts the most pressure.

Breathe and relax. While breathing, try to keep your jaw loose and slightly open to counteract any tendency to clench the teeth. Don't force your breathing. Just breathe gently and easily while you are using the block. If there is discomfort, you may tend to hold your breath—try not to.

In the beginning, do not use the block more than four or five minutes at a time. As your discomfort decreases, gradually increase the amount of time you use the block.

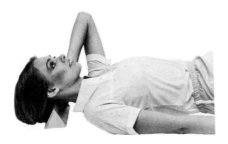

Use the block twice daily until you no longer feel pain. Using the block at regular intervals is most effective. Once each morning and evening is a good routine. Eventually the block will not hurt at all and its use will be pleasant. When the tension has been sufficiently reduced, you need use the block only as a tension detector. Place it under the occiput briefly several times a week to get a tension reading. If it hurts, you know you should use the block regularly again. If it feels fine, your level of neck tension is still low.

If the block is used to excess, soreness may develop. If this occurs, discontinue use until the soreness is gone. Even after all discomfort is gone, it is very important not to leave your head on the block at one place longer than thirty seconds.

The block is not intended as a cure for anything, but as an aid to breaking down tension in the head and neck. It can rid you of discomfort from physical tension in that area. However, for those with severe neck tension, the block will probably not be effective and professional help should be sought (see Appendix).

## 2.

### The Head Push

If you are quite stiff in the neck, try this exercise to increase mobility. Sit or stand in an upright position. Keep your eyes directed straight ahead. Without moving your torso, move your head forward and then backward. Do it as far as you can in both directions without straining. The motion resembles a chicken moving its head and neck. Keep your mouth slightly open to prevent clenching your jaw. Be sure to keep breathing while doing this exercise. Do this five to ten times, two or three times throughout the day.

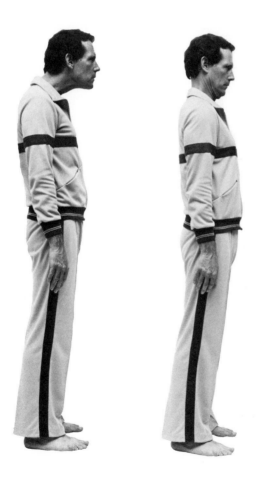

## THE SHOULDERS

All three of the following shoulder exercises are described more fully in Chapter 4.

## 1.

### Arm Circles

Vigorously circle the arm as if pitching a softball (see page 87)

## 2.

### The Shoulder Drop

Raise the shoulders while breathing in, and let them drop with gravity on your exhale. Do it slowly, then fast (see page 72).

## 3.

### Shoulder Rolls

Circle your shoulders vigorously in both directions (see page 72).

## THE ARMS AND HANDS

# 1.

## Towel-Twisting

Roll up a towel and twist it as if you were wringing it out. Try to keep your hands in constant motion. It doesn't matter how slightly they move. Twist for two to four seconds, and then relax. Do this several times in one direction. Then roll the towel the other way and twist it in the opposite direction. Do this four or five times in each direction. Don't hold your breath.

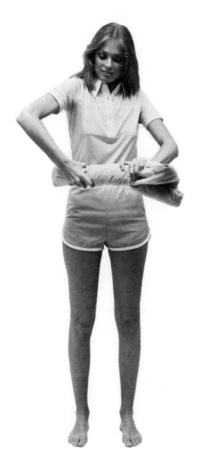

## 2.

### Hand-Shaking

Shake your hands vigorously while moving them out to the side and then above your head, breathing as you move. Shake for as long as you can and as vigorously as you can.

## THE CHEST AND CENTER BACK

### The Large-Ball Chest Release

To do this exercise you need a *soft* rubber ball about 5 inches in diameter. Lie on the floor on your back and place the ball directly under your spine in the center back between your shoulder blades.

Extend your arms up and out to the sides. Breathe and relax for two to four minutes. Then begin circling one arm to the side and above your head freely through space, very slowly, reaching gently out toward the walls and ceiling. Your arms should move as if in slow motion with periodic rests. Circle the other arm in the same way, then move both arms together.

This exercise helps to release tension in the center and upper back, chest, diaphragm, and upper abdomen. It helps you breathe a little more deeply. Do it at least several times a week, for about ten minutes each time.

If you are not too tense, the ball will feel pleasant and there will be no discomfort. Experiment with different sized balls of varying firmness to find the right one for you. If you are very tight, you will need a smaller one or a very soft one.

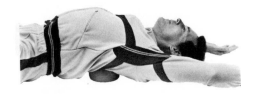

## THE LOWER BACK

1.

### The Pelvic Release

Either lying, sitting, or standing, forcefully tighten the muscles of your buttocks, hold them for a moment, and then let go. Rest for a moment and then try it again. Repeat this five to ten times.

2.

### The Pelvic Swing

Stand with your feet parallel, about 3 or 4 inches apart. Place one hand on your abdomen and the other on your buttocks. Stand upright and bend your knees a little, keeping your heels on the ground. Throughout this exercise your hands will let you know if you are forcefully tightening your abdominal and hip muscles. Tighten them for a moment now, so that your hands can feel the difference.

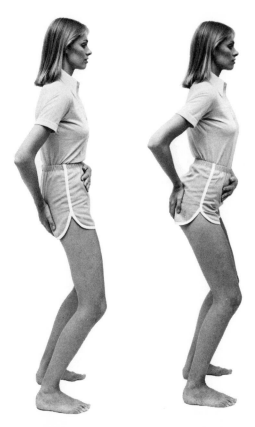

*Phase I.* Keeping your abdominal and buttock muscles as relaxed as possible, gently swing your pelvis as far forward as you can and then as far back as you can. Don't push or tighten.

*Phase II.* See your "sit bones" (the two bones you sit on) as headlights shining down onto the floor beneath you. As you swing your pelvis forward and back, your lights shine a little in front of you and a little in back of you. Perform the movements slowly and easily. Do this ten or fifteen times before taking a break. It should take very little effort.

Be sure to keep your body stationary; there is a tendency to lean forward and back. The pelvis should be able to swing freely. The hamstring muscles and the psoas muscles deep in the abdomen do most of the work. You don't have to forcefully tighten the external muscles to do the action. If it is difficult or hurts when moving in either direction, make smaller movements in that direction, and try to stop before you come to that uncomfortable place.

This exercise is also good for those who get lower-back pain. It helps release tension and is good as a lower-back warm-up exercise.

## THE ENTIRE BACK AND THE HIPS

### The Small-Ball Techniques

The ball techniques for the back and hips work because they increase the tension in a muscle beyond its tolerance level. When this happens, the brain signals the release of some tension and an increase of blood circulation results. If you find any of the ball techniques painful, your back or hips are very tense. Start slowly and build gradually. If you find the techniques too uncomfortable to do on the floor, do them on a bed until your muscles soften up enough to tolerate more pressure. All you need is a small ball the size and firmness of a tennis ball.

## 1.
### The Upper Back

The three techniques that follow work on a muscle group called the erector spinae, which runs from the back of the head through the neck and all the way down the back, flanking both sides of the spine, to where it attaches at the tops of the hip bones.

Place the ball on the floor. Lie on your back so that you are compressing the ball with the muscles between the spine and one shoulder blade. Lie on the ball for a minute or so until you feel your back letting go. Then slowly move the ball by slightly shifting your body in a zigzag fashion, so that the ball moves toward or away from the spine alternately, covering a distance of about 2 inches. Stop at various points along the way when you feel a tight or painful spot. Then try it on the other side. Use the ball through the whole area between the shoulder blade and the spine from the top to the bottom of the shoulder blade, but never run the spine directly over the ball with pressure.

This technique releases tension in the shoulders and upper back. It can be used for general tension and also will help an injured or spasmodic area. You can do it as often as needed. If you like, use two balls simultaneously, one on each side.

2.
## The Center Back

Place the ball under the middle back—that region extending from just below the shoulder blade to the lower end of the rib cage—and move it from side to side slowly on one side of the spine, stopping at various places. Then move over to the other side. Go up and down, and cover the entire center-back area.

You need not limit the exercise to the muscles next to the spine; move out farther to the sides. Make sure you are breathing regularly. In this section of the back, it is sometimes helpful to use two balls at the same time.

This exercise is good for center-back and chest tension. It is especially helpful for those who have difficulty breathing because of chest or diaphragm tension. Do it as often as you like.

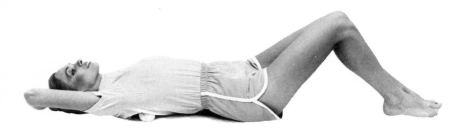

3.

## The Lower Back

Place the ball under your lower back and move it from side to side as in the preceding exercise. Leave the ball in one place for a while, then move it to a new place, covering the whole lower-back area. *Be careful of the spine*. With the ball on the right side of your lower back, raise your right knee toward your chest. This intensifies the pressure. The ball exercise done in this area reduces the tension in the lower back and increases flexibility and blood circulation. It's also good for menstrual cramps and for the lower-back tension that women often experience during pregnancy. Do it as often as needed, but be careful not to use too much pressure, since this is a sensitive area.

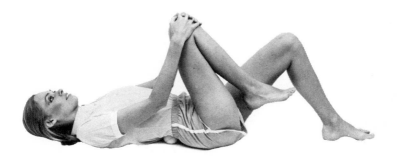

4.
## The Hips

Lie on your back with one knee raised and the sole of your foot on the floor. Place the ball at various places under your hip and slowly lower the raised knee to the side (see photo).

Leave the ball in one position for thirty or forty seconds with your knee lowered; then raise your leg, find a new place for the ball, and repeat. Then do the other hip.

This exercise relieves tension in the hips. Do it as often as necessary. If your hips are quite muscular or have a lot of excess weight, you may need to use a harder ball. A lacrosse ball works well.

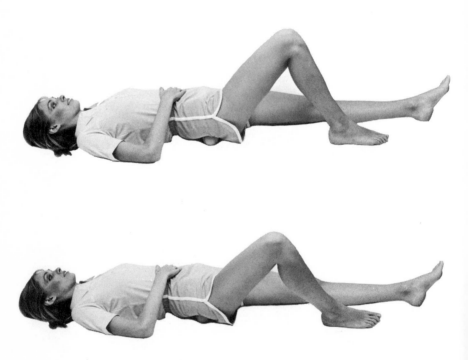

## THE LEGS AND FEET

### 1.

### Stamping

With your shoes on, walk around the house on a carpeted floor or outside on the earth, stamping your feet forcefully into the ground, always maintaining a slightly bent knee on impact. Do this for two or three minutes without stopping.

### 2.

### Foot-Shaking

While sitting, standing, or lying down, forcefully shake one foot at a time for ten to fifteen seconds. Repeat this, alternating three or four times. Be sure to breathe as you do it. Foot-Shaking can also be done as described in the general body warm-up, page 53.

### 3.

### Water Kicking

Lie on your back when you go swimming and kick very forcefully for a minute or two followed by a rest, floating.

### 4.

### Elevating the Legs

Lie on your back on the floor with your lower legs on a chair for five to ten minutes (see page 37).

## THE TOTAL BODY

The Shake-down exercise described below is an excellent full-body relaxation technique. In addition, warm baths, the shower massage, a whirlpool, and a sauna are excellent as regular procedures that will help you to relax (see pages 35–37).

### The Shake-down

Stand with your feet parallel, about a foot apart. Drop your head, resting your chin on your chest. Bend through your spine, one vertebra at a time, as you gradually move your head toward the floor. As you are doing this, allow your knees to bend slightly. Stop when your head is in front of your knees and the tips of your fingers are touching the floor. Hang in this position with your arms totally relaxed. Take a few deep breaths and gently shake your shoulders.

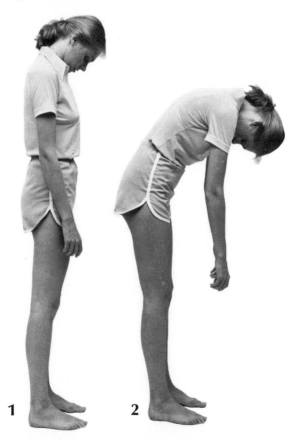

1          2

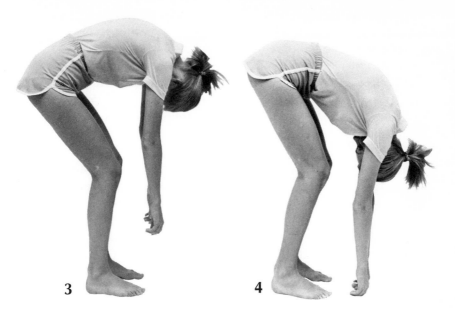

3          4

Now reverse the process. Beginning from the base of your spine, straighten your back, vertebra by vertebra. Don't lift your head until you are fully erect. Do this exercise several times varying the speed, but never fast.

Once you've become comfortable with the Shake-down, try this variation. Remain in the position where your fingers touch the ground and take a few deep breaths. Now lift just your head and look at the floor in front of your feet. Then drop your head suddenly and let it swing forward and back until it stops by itself. When you drop your head, it should move only by the force of gravity. Then, as in the original version of this exercise, slowly roll back up until you're standing upright. Do five or six sets of both variations. You can alternate them, if you like.

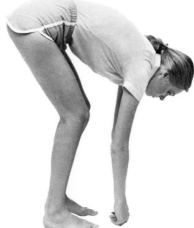

## TOTAL-BODY IMAGE RELAXATION

We rarely take the time to exercise the powers of our mind in order to relax and reduce tension. Concentrating on an image takes your mind off of everything else, and this alone helps the brain and nervous system to slow you down. Relaxation imagery cannot get rid of years of excess tension, but the exercises that follow can help you to relax up to the maximum of your present capability.

To prepare yourself for these relaxing images, lie down on your back in a quiet place. It may help to place pillows under your head and knees. Take the phone off the hook and tell people not to disturb you. Image relaxation can also be practiced while floating on your back in the water.

You can alter these total-body relaxation images to match your own experience if you wish. After you select one of the following relaxation-imagery exercises and read it through three or four times, put the book down. Close your eyes, become aware of your breathing, and relax. Give yourself time to settle before you begin, and try to maintain a strong picture of the image in your mind's eye as if it were projected on a large movie screen right before you.

If you have a friend with a pleasant, relaxing voice, have the image read to you very slowly, with a long pause between each sentence or idea. Otherwise, it is a good idea to make a tape recording of the images you plan to use. Make sure to read them slowly, allowing plenty of time between thoughts.*

Essentially what you are trying to do is imagine yourself in a relaxed place or situation or give yourself an image that contains movement which will allow you to let go of some tension. Your brain controls every single muscle in your body. If you can learn to have it work for you, you can relax anywhere, anytime.

*A selection of prerecorded relaxation tapes can be purchased from Relaxation Tools, Inc., P.O. Box 1045, New York, N.Y. 10025.

## 1.

### Ocean Water

Imagine yourself on a beautiful beach. It's pleasantly hot and the sky is a deep blue. There is a sweet, cool breeze caressing your body as you walk, carrying your softly inflated rubber raft into the clear blue-green sea. You lie down on your back on the raft and your body sinks slightly into the water. The sun is warm and your body sways in the wake of the water's movement. Your breathing deepens unconsciously as your body relaxes to the rocking of the waves. Your arms begin to drift into the water and let go. It's as if the sea were drawing the tension out of them. Your shoulders release as their heaviness drifts into your arms and out your hands in the refreshing, cool water. As your body temperature adjusts to the water, it feels deliciously warm.

Feel the hot sun as it beams down on your forehead, your nose, your cheeks, and your mouth. It drains out the heaviness in you. Gently your head slips back off the raft and floats into the water. Your scalp is bathed in coolness—which then turns pleasantly warm—sifting out your busy thoughts. Your head feels buoyant and supported by the deep, resilient liquid warmth. The feeling of the sun's hotness is now upon your neck, which releases and relaxes as your mouth drops quietly open to allow more breath to enter and to leave you.

The raft seems to dissolve and your legs float apart as if by someone else's will and they slide into the soft water. They begin to tingle as their sweat is washed away by the coolness. They relax as they drift and melt into the water. Your legs feel the pull of the current and after a moment they feel as if they are getting longer and longer.

There is a wavy buoyancy under your back and hips as they appear to widen and sink deeper into the water. The water seems even warmer now as your whole body merges with the sea and feels weightless and at ease. You drift now to the sounds of the clouds, the sun, and the sky. You relax and let go as you feel the pleasure of the heat in your skin. Enjoy yourself.

## 2.

### The Blue Light

My favorite tension-releasing color is blue, which is why I call this exercise "the Blue Light." Close your eyes and focus on *your* favorite color, whatever it may be. Picture your color as a warm, glowing light about 3 inches in diameter. See the light hover above your head so that it shines right down onto your face. Feel its warmth dissolving your tension. Now focus the light on your forehead. Move it back and forth across your forehead, vacuuming the tension out of your head.

Take the light to the very top of your head. Move it through your hair gently and slowly. Wherever it shines, the tension dissolves. Now move it above your eyes and focus it there for a few minutes. Now shine the light on your jaw and into your mouth. Now deepen your breathing without forcing, and feel the light shining through to the back of your neck. After a while, shine the light on your chest. Picture it expanding until it illuminates your entire chest. Imagine your chest getting warm and its tension dissolving as the light travels downward.

Feel the warmth spreading through your body, to the upper and center back. Do it very slowly. Don't rush. Next, slowly move a narrowed beam down one arm—the upper arm first, then the lower arm and hand. Now move to the other arm.

Picture the light dissolving the tension in your abdomen. Let the light grow and shine through to the lower back. Slowly continue this process down through the pelvis, thighs, knees, lower legs, ankles, feet, and toes. The Blue Light should take between five and ten minutes.

3.

## Sand Streams in a Hammock

See yourself on a beautiful, deserted beach lying in a luxurious hammock tied between two palm trees. You are in the sun or the shade, whichever you prefer. Imagine your body is filled with fine sand. There are thousands of small holes along the entire undersurface of your body. The sand begins to trickle slowly out of the holes in your feet and lower legs. It falls through the hammock and onto the beach. After a few moments the sand begins to stream out in a steady flow. A warm breeze begins to blow and the hammock swings and sways quietly between the trees. The sand flows out in a steady stream from your thighs and hips now. As the sand empties from your lower body, you perceive a lightness coming over you, as if the weight has dropped out of you. Now the sand starts to pour from your lower back and then your center back, taking with it all the tension. Then the sand begins to pour out of your upper back and shoulders.

Move the sand flow slowly from place to place throughout your body, the slower the better. The fine sand streams out of you and into the wind, and as you rock to the sounds of the ocean breeze, become aware of where you feel heavy or tense. This awareness should surface now that you are more relaxed. When you feel a blocked or tight place, let the sand flow from it until it empties some more.

# 7

# STRETCHING

The word *flexibility* technically refers to the range of movement of the bones within a joint. Joint flexibility is more limited in adults than in children because their ligaments and bones are fully developed. Flexibility in joints is also dependent on the muscles and tendons.

The relationship between ligaments, tendons, and muscle elasticity is actually very simple to understand. Your ligaments hold your bones together and have a microscopically small amount of elasticity. This means that if they are extended or stretched beyond their normal maximum length, they will not return to their original state. When a ligament becomes permanently stretched, it is more prone to injury because the joint it holds together is not as secure and stable as it once was. When you dislocate your shoulder more than once, the ligaments that hold it in place become permanently stretched out, and this increases the possibility that the shoulder will dislocate again and again.

Muscles are attached to bones by tough, fibrous connective tissues called tendons. Tendons are only slightly more elastic than ligaments in returning to their original length after being stretched. If you stretch your tendons instead of your muscles it often results in strained and injured tendons.

Only muscles are elastic and tend to return to their original length. A muscle at rest has a particular length, referred to as its "resting length."

At any given time there is a limit to how far a muscle can be stretched. That is its present maximum length. When you do stretching exercises over a period of time, the resting length of the muscle fibers increases. If you stretch properly and consistently, your muscles will remain in a new, more lengthened or stretched position. If you don't stretch regularly, your muscles will return to their original length.

The term *flexibility* is often applied to muscles as well as to joints. It means that the muscles are very elastic and pliable, stretching easily. If your muscles are relaxed and stretched properly, your maximum joint flexibility is available to you.

The capacity for full range of movement is an advantage in avoiding injury. Most people don't realize how flexible their joints and ligaments can be. Their muscles are seldom loose enough to allow the full movement range of the joints. With maximum stretch your body develops the ability to move in a wider range without danger. Your muscles will not try to stop you when you move suddenly into an extreme position, such as a lunge to catch a falling dish or a fly ball.

People who have very limited flexibility in their joints should work gently and consistently to obtain maximum flexibility in their muscles. This takes considerable time and effort. Most people tense their muscles, stretch forcefully, and end up stretching their ligaments or tendons. This gives them the appearance of being stretched out, with all of the dangers and none of the benefits. You must stretch your muscles, not your ligaments or tendons.

## THE STRETCH REFLEX

The most important concept in learning how to stretch is the "stretch reflex," the body's automatic protective mechanism against severe injury and abuse. Whenever a muscle is stretched too quickly or with a lot of force, a message is sent from the brain to the muscle to contract instantly so it is not injured. *Stretching can be effective only if it is done slowly and gently.* You can't stretch a muscle that's in a contraction; it's a contradiction. It's like someone standing outside your front door trying to open it with all his might while you stand inside and use all your force in keeping it closed. When you stretch this way, you do an awful lot of work, but you don't really get anywhere.

The best positions for stretching are lying down or sitting, because the parts of the body you want to stretch should not be bearing weight.

When you stand, your legs are holding you up. In order to keep you standing, the muscle fibers in the legs are contracting. If they were relaxed, you would fall down. When you try to stretch your leg muscles in a standing position, you are attempting to elongate a muscle that you are actively contracting in order to stand up. You are working against yourself. If you stand when you stretch, you often end up invoking the stretch reflex. When you bounce up and down in any position or vigorously force a muscle to lengthen, the stretch reflex also occurs.

## TENSION DECREASES FLEXIBILITY

An additional factor that can limit your ability to gain stretch and your natural range of movement is chronic tension. A muscle cannot attain its maximum length unless it can relax. There are two approaches to stretching, depending upon how tense you are. If you're quite tense, progress will be difficult unless you loosen up the muscles first. You have to learn how to relax your muscles before you can stretch effectively. To do this I recommend the relaxation techniques found in Chapter 6. Another good way to prepare for stretching is to take a warm bath just before you stretch. If you are fairly relaxed, but somewhat inflexible, regularly do the stretching series suggested at the end of this chapter. This will help your muscles reach their maximum length capacity fairly easily.

## HOW TO STRETCH

In order to tell whether you are stretching correctly, you must be able to tell where the action is happening. Pay attention to precisely where the pulling sensation is. You should feel the pull in the meaty part of the muscle. If the sensation is felt near a joint only, you are stretching the ligament or tendon. Always try to do the exercise so that you feel it throughout the bulk of the muscle. You may have to bend or straighten your leg a little more, or you may have to try a different exercise. Don't sacrifice your joint stability by stretching your ligaments in order to gain greater freedom of joint movement.

An important rule to follow is: *Never stretch unless you are thoroughly warmed up.* When your muscles are warm and surging with blood, the tissues are literally more pliable. It's similar to what happens when you put honey in the refrigerator—it gets stiff and pours slowly. When you heat it up, it becomes more liquified, and in a sense stretches out, pouring more easily. Your muscles work in much the same way. When your body is cold, it resists stretching and will invoke the stretch reflex very quickly. Any stretching that occurs will be at the joints rather than the muscles. This kind of stretch won't last and can make you more prone to injury.

It is best to stretch after your run, your game, or your exercise class. You should have a minimum of five to ten minutes of very vigorous activity before stretching. If you want to stretch at home, do the general body warm-up, the lower-body warm-up, run in place, or dance to your favorite record for five to ten minutes first.

As a general rule, and in all of the stretches that follow, *the best way to stretch is to gently ease your body into the stretched position.* Relax, breathe, and stay there for ten to fifteen seconds. Don't pull or work to stretch farther; simply keep breathing. Let your body adjust slowly. You might stretch farther next time. If the stretch is one-sided—that is, one leg at a time—then proceed to the other side. If it is a two-sided stretch—that is, sitting and hanging forward stretching both hamstrings at once—rest for a few moments before you try it again.

Don't push yourself to pain. Stretch to the point where you feel a pulling sensation *throughout* the muscle, not at the ends near the joint. The farthest you should go is mild discomfort. As you become more stretched, that discomfort should disappear.

As it becomes easier to stay in the stretched position for fifteen seconds, begin to increase the length of time that you relax into the stretched position. Work your way to thirty seconds, making sure to breathe regularly throughout. After a month or two of regular stretching, you should be able to stay in many of the positions for up to a full minute. Remember: Don't bounce and never force. Stretching is only effective after you have fully warmed up and is especially good to do following your work-out.

The amount of stretching you have to do to maintain your new maximum length capacity depends upon the level of tension in your body. The more stretch you desire, the more frequently you have to stretch. To maintain an increased flexibility, you should stretch a minimum of three times a week. If you're a professional—a dancer, for instance—and have to maintain unusual amounts of flexibility, you'll need to stretch five to six times a week.

## WHAT TO STRETCH

We generally need to have the greatest muscle flexibility in the parts of our body that must support our weight. There is a constant demand for muscle contraction in the lower body just to hold us up. This can lead to a buildup of tension and a shortening of the resting length of the muscle. Thus, most people feel the need to stretch out the muscles of the lower back and the backs of the legs, commonly called the hamstrings. The front thigh muscles, or quadriceps, are among the strongest single muscles in our body. It is often good to stretch them just to let them recover from the constant demands of bearing weight. Stretching these muscles will improve the efficiency of their contraction, by increasing their length, and will increase their range of motion.

## THE STRETCHING EXERCISES

Do the stretching exercises on the following pages that feel the best. You may want to do only a few of the stretches for your body's particular needs, or you may want to do them all, several times a week. The calf and hamstring stretches get progressively harder. Stick with the first of each of these for a week or two before going on to the next. Remember, the criterion for a good stretch for you is that you feel the pull in the middle of the muscle, not at either end.

After you have learned all of the stretches, I suggest you do them regularly after an extensive warm-up or workout. At the end of this chapter I have arranged the stretches in a series that I think is the best possible progression for a total stretching program. I have varied the parts of the body so as to alternately rest each one and to achieve maximum effect. After you have learned all the stretches thoroughly, write them out on a 3 x 5 index card and put the card in your pocket or your bag so that you can refer it to when you need it.

The last two stretches, for the hand and forearm, are an optional addition. They are good to do in the middle of a handball game, a tennis game, or any racket sport. If you have had trouble with your hand or wrist or have tennis elbow, it is good to do them after you have warmed up thoroughly and volleyed for five minutes or so.

## THE CALVES

## 1.

### The Towel Calf Stretch

Sit on the floor with your legs extended, a foot or so apart. Fold a bath towel lengthwise and hold it at the ends. Place it around the ball of your foot as if in you were in a saddle stirrup. With your knee straight but not locked, gently pull the towel toward you by leaning back until you feel your calf muscles stretch a little. Stay in this position for ten to fifteen seconds, then release it. If you don't feel the stretch in the belly of the muscle, bend your knee a little at a time until you do. The stretch should not hurt. If it does, don't pull so hard or hold it as long. Coax it, and you'll win. Push it, and you'll lose.

Alternate right and left for two to four sets. In several weeks, when it feels easier, gradually increase the pull and the time you maintain it to thirty to forty seconds.

Always breathe and relax as you do it. Try not to let the top of the pelvis fall backward as you stretch. If it does, you lose the leverage for stretching the calf. Bending the other leg is often helpful, especially for men. It is best to stretch the calf with the calf and knee supported by the ground. If you do it in the air, it is easy to lock the knee and therefore put stress on the structures surrounding the knee.

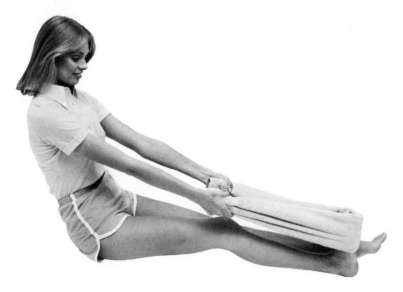

2.

## The Wall Lean

Stand 3 to 5 feet away from a wall. Make sure your feet are parallel and 2 to 3 inches apart. Place your hands on the wall in front of you at shoulder height. Now bend your elbows until both your forearms are resting against the wall. The top of your head just above your forehead may also touch the wall. Try to support your weight with your forearms and head.

It's important to locate the distance from the wall that is best for you. Your position is correct when your feet are as far from the wall as possible with your heels flat on the floor and your knees straight but not locked. While leaning, adjust your feet until they're placed at the right distance to feel a stretch throughout your calf muscles.

Try to keep your body in a straight diagonal, being careful not to let your pelvis stick out in back or drop toward the floor. A stable position makes it much easier to measure your progress.

Remain in the Wall Lean position for ten to fifteen seconds. Then walk toward the wall and then relax for a minute before you try it again. This exercise is fairly intense, so only do it three or four times. During the next month or two, gradually increase your distance from the wall and the time that you hold the stretch. It can be held for up to a minute. You can accent one leg at a time, but *don't* bounce.

The Wall Lean should not be done unless you are very warmed up, and only after you can do the Towel Calf Stretch fairly easily. Do it slowly. Don't force it.

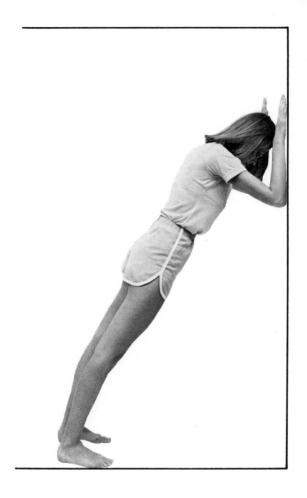

## THE HAMSTRINGS

3.

### The Towel Hamstring Stretch

Lie on your back with a bath towel looped around the back of your lower leg behind your ankle or around your heel, with your knee slightly bent. As you do this stretch, vary the amount of bend in your knee. Gently pull your foot toward your head, while keeping your leg as relaxed as possible. Keep your elbows close to your body to minimize tension in the shoulders. Hold it for ten to fifteen seconds, then release it. As it becomes easier for you, the leg will be more comfortable in a more straightened position. As you change the bend in the knee, you will feel the stretch more in the upper, middle, or lower sections of the hamstrings.

As you do the stretch, be sure to keep your leg pointing straight ahead; don't let it turn out. Remember to avoid positions where you feel the stretch only at the extreme ends of the muscle. Vary the angle of your knee. As you become more stretched, you may move the towel toward the heel for additional leverage. If you have very flexible hamstrings, it may be easier for you to use your hands to hold onto your ankle.

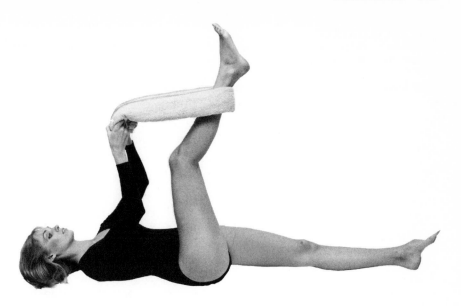

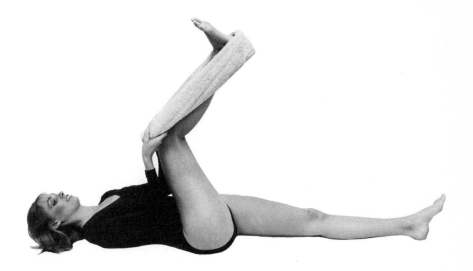

4.

## The Hamstring Floor Lean

If you can easily sit on the floor with your back upright and your legs straight out in front of you, without pulling or straining sensations in your back or in the front of your hip joints, you are sufficiently flexible to do this exercise. If not, wait until you have done the Towel Hamstring Stretch for a month or so before you try it. If you suffer from lower back pain this is not a good stretch for you. Stick to the Towel Hamstring Stretch.

Sit on the floor with your legs straight in front of you, about 18 inches apart. With your arms dangling in front of you, leading with the top of your head and curving your spine, let the weight of your body fall gently forward. Relax your legs and breathe regularly. Don't worry if your legs tend to bend a little. Stay in this position for about thirty seconds, then straighten up. Try this several times. Now bend forward again and this time lift your hands so they are just off the floor. Breathe and relax. This adds 10 or 15 pounds of weight to stretch you a little farther.

After you have done this for several days, or if you find it too easy, lift a book in your hands as you relax forward. As time goes by, lift a slightly heavier book. Use a 2-inch phone book, with 5 pounds as the maximum weight. As you get good at this, bring your legs closer and closer together. This makes the stretch more and more intense, but only do it if you can do so with ease.

Do not flex your feet and try to stretch your calves at the same time.

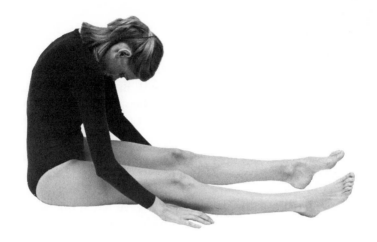

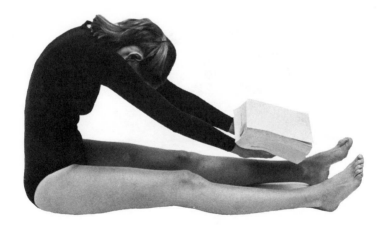

## THE QUADRICEPS

### 5.

### The Front-Lying Quadriceps Stretch

Sit on your right hip, with your legs bent. Take hold of the top of your left foot with your left hand. Now slide down so that you are lying face down with your head turned to the left. Bring your bent leg in line with your straight one. It will tend to remain out to the side. Now draw your heel gently toward the center of your buttocks, as far as it will go easily.

Resist the temptation to bounce your foot. Hold it for five to ten seconds to begin with, gradually increasing to 50 to 60 seconds over a month. Breathe regularly and imagine the front of your thigh getting longer. Never do both legs at the same time. When in this position, try not to lift your pelvis off the floor. Allowing the front of the pelvis to come off the floor strains the lower back and minimizes the amount of stretch you get.

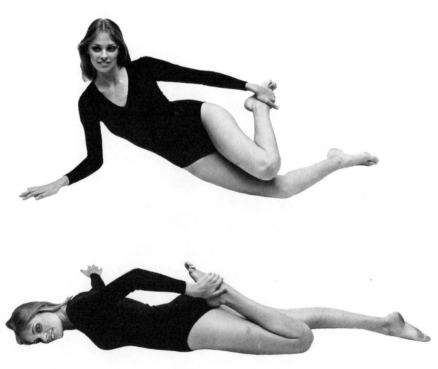

## THE BACK

6.

### The Sitting Back Stretch

It is especially difficult to isolate the lower back for stretching. In order to effectively stretch the back, you must keep your pelvis upright. Place your hand under your buttocks and feel for your "sit bones," the bones you sit on, at the bottom of your pelvis. There is one on each side. Rock from side to side so that you feel them and become aware of where they are. Now slump in your chair and feel how you roll backward off of them. In order to remain squarely on your sit bones, you have to keep your pelvis upright. If your pelvis slumps backward, you only stretch the upper back. If the top of your pelvis hangs forward and your belly hangs out, you compress your hip joints and stretch your hamstring muscles.

To do this exercise, you need to have a chair that's the right height for you. (To determine your correct chair height, see page 38.) Sit in the chair with your feet parallel and in front of you.

**6A.** Sit on the edge of the chair with your feet 18 inches to 2 feet apart. Fold your hands and place them behind your neck at the base of your skull. Keeping your body erect, allow your head to fall forward and your upper back to relax. Remain in this position for thirty seconds. Breathe and relax. Now come up and rest. This stretches the upper back.

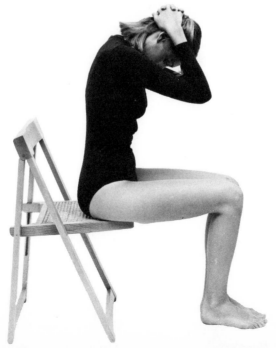

**6B.** Repeat the exercise, only this time allow your back to round forward several inches, so that you feel the pull in the center portion of your back. Make sure your pelvis remains upright. This will be different for each individual, depending on how flexible your back muscles are. You can control exactly where the stretch occurs by how far you bend forward.

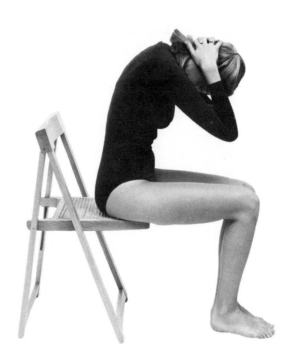

**6C.** This time, round forward even more until you feel the pull in your lower back. Make sure you bend at the waist and not at the hip joint. You do not have to go down very far toward the floor. Your elbows will probably not get much lower than your knees.

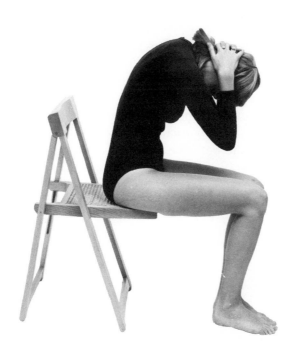

## THE WAIST

7.

### The Progressive Side Stretch

Sit on an armless chair, with your feet flat on the floor and parallel, about 18 inches apart. Imagine your body lifting upward as you bend to the right. Let your arms hang to the side as you reach up and out with the top of your head. Try to maintain a lifted feeling if you can, and don't let your pelvis hyperextend or come off the chair. Breathe regularly as you move. Don't hold this stretch; simply go as far as you can to the right and then to the left. As this becomes easier, add more weight to the stretch by placing your hands behind your head and repeat as before. You can make the stretch even more intense later by raising your hands above your head. Keep your elbows slightly bent as you lean to the side. If on a particular day you feel strain, only do the stretch the easy way. Alternate five times on each side.

This exercise can be done standing, but make sure not to let your pelvis shift to the side.

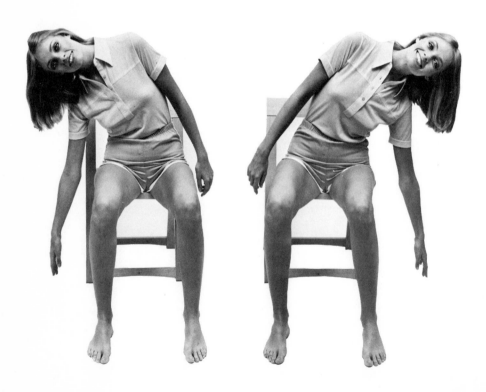

## THE ADDUCTORS

8.

### The Bent-Knee Adductor Stretch

Lie on your back, fold your knees to your chest, and take hold of the insides of your knees so they fall open toward the floor. Your thighs should be at a right angle to your body. Don't pull your knees up high, and don't try to force them open toward the floor; just relax and let gravity stretch you. Hold this position for ten to fifteen seconds only, then close your legs and relax for a few moments before trying it again. As your stretch increases and you find the exercise easier to do, increase your time slowly until you can hold it for a full minute.

The Bent-Knee Adductor Stretch is not for you if you feel the stretch in the tendon near the groin or in the ligament inside the hip joint. This results from a previous weakening of the tendon or ligament structure. It can also be caused by contracting your muscles to hold the legs up, instead of letting them go. If this happens, try the Wall Adductor Stretch instead. In that exercise the wall helps to support the legs, allowing you to relax and stretch the belly of the adductor muscles.

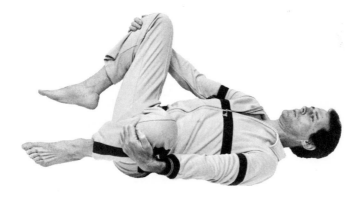

## 9.

## The Wall Adductor Stretch

Find an empty wall about 6 feet wide that you can use regularly without having to move much furniture. Lie on your back on the floor with your legs raised against the wall. Move in close so that your legs are at a 90-degree angle to your body and your buttocks are touching the wall. Keeping your knees slightly bent, slowly open your legs as far as they will go without forcing them. Adjust the bend in your knees to an angle that lets you feel stretch throughout the inner thigh muscles. Allow gravity to do the work for you. Stay in this position as long as you feel comfortable, up to five minutes. You can read, talk on the phone, or breathe and relax. Place a pillow under the back of your pelvis if it's uncomfortable.

In both of the adductor exercises, the normal weight of your legs gently and gradually pulls them down, stretching your inner thigh muscles.

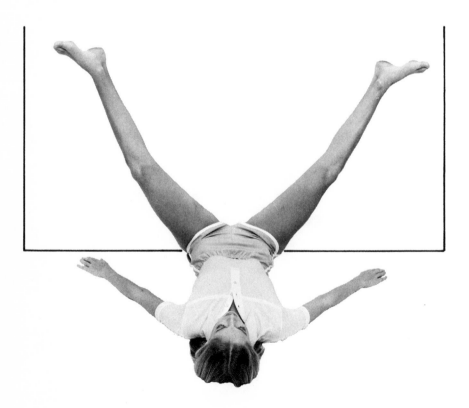

**THE NECK**

## 10.

### The Neck Stretch

Clasp your hands behind your neck and allow your head to fall forward, keeping your spine vertical. This can be done while sitting or standing. Breathe and relax in this position for ten to fifteen seconds. Then bring your head upright and rest for a moment. Repeat as before, only this time rest your hands an inch higher, at the base of your skull. This gives you the maximum stretch. Only do it this way if it feels good. The additional force might cause you discomfort, so listen to what your body says.

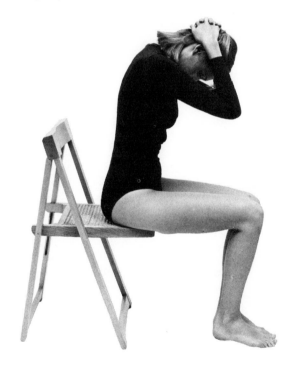

## THE HANDS AND FOREARMS

# 11.

### The Wrist Stretch

With your left hand, grip the back of your right hand just below the wrist. The thumb is on the inside and the other fingers, except for the index finger, are on the outside. Hold your hands in front of your abdomen. Now, stretch your wrist by lifting your hands slowly up toward your chest. Be sure to keep your elbows stationary. Hold them there for several seconds. Stop before you feel any real discomfort. Lower your hands and repeat. Do this six to eight times with each hand. Repeat this sequence two or three times.

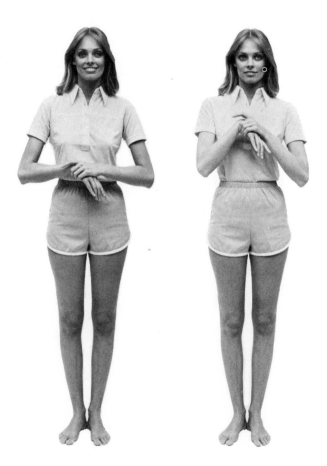

## 12.

### The Palm Press

Begin with your hands in front of your neck, in a prayer position. Press your palms and fingers into each other and moderately push your hands together as you draw them downward. Move them vertically down toward your abdomen as far as you can, allowing the heels of your hands to separate slightly. Hold your hands here for several seconds before returning them to their original position. After a while, you'll be able to draw your hands lower and lower. Rest briefly between each movement. Slowly increase the number of Palm Presses up to a maximum of thirty.

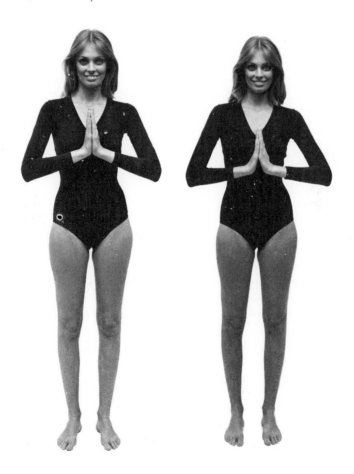

## THE CHEST

# 13.

## The Large-Ball Chest Release

This technique is described on page 122.

## THE TOTAL BODY

# 14.

## The Shake-down

This technique is described on page 130.

### THE STRETCH SERIES

1.   The Shake-down
2.   The Towel Calf Stretch
3.   The Towel Hamstring Stretch
     A.  On Calf
     B.  On Heel
4.   The Front-Lying Quadriceps Stretch
5.   The Hamstring Floor Lean
     A.  Arms Lifted
     B.  With a Book
6.   The Bent-Knee Adductor Stretch
                    *or*
     The Wall Adductor Stretch
7.   The Neck Stretch
8.   The Sitting Back Stretch
9.   The Progressive Side Stretch
10.  The Wall Lean
11.  The Large-Ball Chest Release

### THE HAND AND FOREARM STRETCHES

1.   The Wrist Stretch
2.   The Palm Press

# 8

# STRENGTH

Strength in the broadest scope is physical power that is active and protective at the same time. When we engage in sports and exercise, we are constantly asking our muscles to meet certain demands. Strength refers to the ability of our muscles to contract in order to perform an action. When a muscle contracts over a certain distance, it produces a specific amount of work. If you simply increase the demand on the muscles gradually, you will get stronger.

The concept of strength is often confused with the concept of endurance. The difference is that endurance involves the factor of time while strength does not. Strength refers only to the ability to perform an action. Endurance refers to how long or how many times the action can be performed.

*Tension dilutes strength.* In a chronically tense muscle, some or all of the fibers are constantly contracted, even when "at rest." A tense muscle has to work extra hard in order to perform. It gets wider and bulkier, becoming hard and rocklike and often developing knots and bulges. When your muscles are kept active and relatively tension-free, they contract more efficiently when performing an action. They are supple and firm, but with resilience rather than hardness, and they can let go completely when at rest. Thus, more of your potential strength and energy is available to you.

You do not need to have large, bulging muscles in order to be strong. Many dancers and gymnasts attain incredible amounts of strength without looking like weight lifters. The excess muscle bulk associated with incredible strength is also an indicator of excess muscle tension. It is possible to become strong with or without tension. Tension is not necessary for strength. Be careful when you are building strength that you aren't also building tension.

## HOW MUCH STRENGTH DO YOU NEED?

Your body begins to build strength from the moment you're able to move. Most people build and maintain the amount of strength they need simply by moving. Being active beyond your daily routine will automatically add to your existing strength capacity. This additional strength increases your fitness, eases the burden of your daily routine, and supplies you with a reservoir of surplus strength for unusually demanding situations.

There are different ideas about how much strength a person actually needs and how to go about building it. Some people want to develop as much strength as they possibly can in order to improve the appearance of their bodies rather than out of concern for their general health. If you regard strength-building as a series of isolated exercises unrelated to your daily activities, such as weight lifting, for example, you may end up building muscles that grossly exceed what is required for natural functioning. Straining or overburdening the muscles will produce both excess muscle bulk and chronic tension at the same time, thereby decreasing your efficiency. Overdeveloping the muscles will also inhibit your full range of movement.

Your body does not require excess amounts of strength to function normally and efficiently. If you are fairly active, you probably have just enough extra strength to make your daily routine easy and to keep you from tiring should you have to exert yourself a little more than usual. If you are thinking about taking up a new sport or activity, it's a good idea to build up your strength in the appropriate areas before you begin. For example, it's a good idea to jog or do thigh-strengthening exercises a few months before you begin skiing. After you have acquired enough strength for your new activity, you won't need to do strength-building exercises anymore.

## HOW TO BUILD STRENGTH

Building strength is a relatively simple process. You just have to use your muscles more than you do now — it's that easy. If you increase the work load on a muscle or muscle group, your strength will increase. If you do this slowly and gradually, you will build a fluid, active, and mobile strength that will protect you as it works for you.

How you do strength-building exercises is almost more important than the particular exercises you choose to do. Constantly straining and pushing to the point of fatigue is destructive. You can be accumulating chronic tension, and laying the groundwork for serious injury.

Increasing the demand on your muscles too quickly or with too many repetitions also endangers the body. The muscles become fatigued, overly tense, and lose flexibility. This can impair your neurological responses and reaction time.

Building strength ought to be a painless, gradual process. Even the mild soreness and stiffness that comes with a new activity should be infrequent. Painless strength-building is a strange concept, and many people think it's impossible. Few people know how to build strength in this painless way, but it's really quite easy once you learn how to do it.

*Maintaining a balance between strength and mobility should be your goal.* Give your muscles ample time to recover during and after a strenuous effort. You begin to lose the ability to build strength after you do a strenuous activity more than two or three times in a row because the muscle begins to fatigue. Do only a couple of strenuous movements or five or six moderate ones before alternating sides. Switch sides often, or rest in between movements. It's better to alternate sides than to keep repeating the same exercises on one side. For example, do five sets of four alternating sides, instead of two sets of ten. It's also a good idea to alternate exercises.

Work slowly and gradually. Don't sacrifice mobility in order to gain strength. Always keep in mind this general rule: *Don't strain!* You should feel a mild stress and that is all.

## CHOOSING STRENGTH-BUILDING
## EXERCISES SUITED FOR YOU

People need different things from an exercise program. Unfortunately, it is not always easy to find the right exercise for you. How you feel while doing a specific exercise isn't necessarily a good barometer of what is appropriate for you. Practically any exercise will make you feel better for a while because it temporarily increases your blood circulation and your breathing rate. So your short-term feelings don't always tell you if an exercise is right for you. Therefore, it's important to know how to judge your exercise needs.

The strengthening exercises in this chapter are designed to build strength without strain. They are not extremely strenuous and can be done easily. But this is not a general strengthening program for everyone. Carefully select the exercises to meet your individual needs by using the results from your fitness profile tests. If you have a chronic injury that is constantly flaring up under stress, carefully choose your exercises accordingly. If an exercise makes you strain, you're not ready for it yet. There will be a suggested number of times to repeat each exercise, but this will change as your strength increases.

The strength-building exercises that follow are intended to be used to help you get started in a new activity. They can also be used to recondition your body while you recover from an injury. They build up muscles that have been weakened through injury and inactivity, or that were previously weak. They allow you to reenter your sport or exercise program with less chance of injury. These exercises are also intended to get you ready after a break from athletic activity, and they can give you a good head start in new activities which require different muscular strength. Lastly, these exercises prepare you for a seasonal sport. For example, before hitting the ski slopes you should spend a month doing leg-strengthening exercises to regain the appropriate muscular strength necessary for skiing.

Here are several guidelines for building efficient strength while maintaining the fluidity of your body.

1. Only use strength-building exercises to help you get started in a new activity or during rehabilitation from an injury.
2. Whenever possible, build strength by doing the activity you wish to do. Static exercises such as isometrics and others which do not involve much movement are not as effective.
3. Stop doing strength-building exercises when you have sufficient strength to perform well and instead play tennis or run or dance or perform some other pleasurable physical activity to maintain your strength.

4. *Always* warm up thoroughly before you begin your strength-building program.
5. Begin slowly, and gradually increase your output during each session and over several months.
6. *Never* hold your breath when you do any strength-building exercises. Breathe through your open mouth as well as through your nose.
7. Lastly, please remember, *If it hurts, don't do it!*

## THE FEET AND LOWER LEGS

# 1.

### Ankle Flexion

Do this exercise sitting down. Lift your foot off the floor with your knee slightly bent. Point and flex the foot more forcefully than you did in the warm-ups. Hold each position for a count of two. Make sure to keep the foot centered in line with the knee. Complete two or three sets with one foot before doing an equal number with the other. Repeat this sequence two or three times. After this becomes easy, try it with your leg straight.

## 2.

### The Elbow-Knee Lean

Sit in a chair of the proper height (see page 38) with your feet flat on the floor. To find the proper starting position, rise onto the ball of your left foot. Adjust your leg until the lower leg is at a 90-degree angle to the floor, as in the second photo. Remain in this position and lower your heel. Now place your right elbow on your thigh just above your right knee, leaning your weight into the lower leg. Slowly raise your heel until you are high on the ball of your foot. Then slowly lower it, while continuing to lean your weight into the lower leg. Do this two or three times with one leg before switching to the other. Do two or three sets.

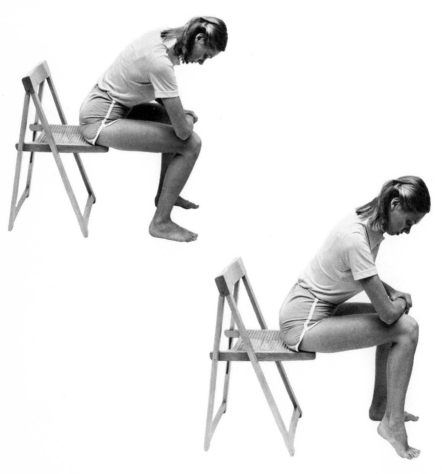

## 3.

### Bent-Knee Heel Raises

Stand with your feet parallel, 3 to 4 inches apart. In order to keep your balance, hold onto a doorknob or a chair. Bend your knees slightly, then slowly rise onto the balls of your feet. Rise up as high as you can without discomfort, keeping your knees bent. Stay in this position for up to five to ten seconds. Then slowly return your heels to the floor and resume standing upright. Relax before attempting the exercise again. Initially, do the exercise five times. Increase the number by one each day until you reach a maximum of fifteen.

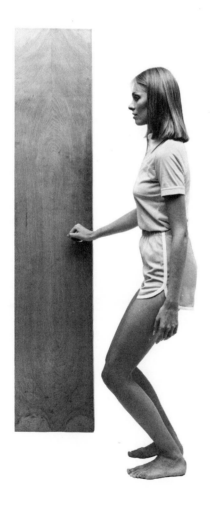 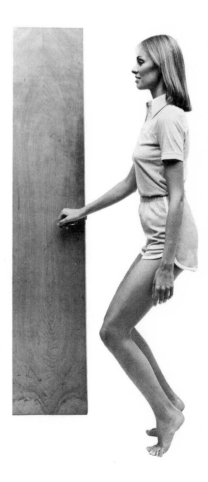

## THE THIGHS

## 1.

### Side-Lying Thigh Lifts

Lie on the floor on your left side with both knees slightly bent. Place your right hand on the floor in front of your chest to stabilize you. Lift your right leg about a foot into the air and then place it back down in the starting position. Do this two to five times, stopping when you begin to tire—it's harder than it looks. Then roll over to the other side and repeat. Alternate several times, stopping each time as you begin to tire.

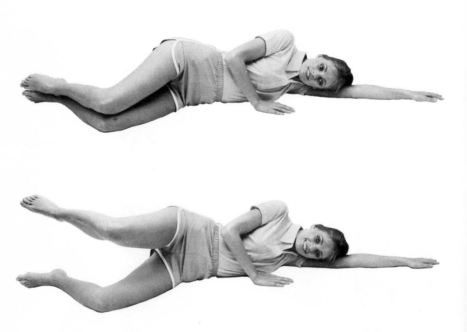

## 2.

### Side-Lying Leg Swings

Begin in the same position as in the previous exercise. With your knee slightly bent, swing your top leg forward and back, keeping it parallel to the floor. Be sure to keep the hand in front of your chest securely on the floor to prevent your body from tipping. Move your leg forward and back to the limits of your range without strain, swinging at a moderate tempo. Do six to ten swings, then roll over to the other side.

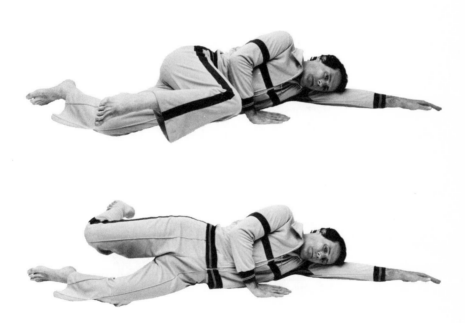

3.

## Thigh Rotation

Begin in the side-lying position. Lift your top leg 6 inches off the floor. While holding it there, rotate the entire leg so that your knee cap turns toward the ceiling. Then rotate the leg inward as far as it will go. Do this three to five times without putting the leg down. Then return your leg to the starting position and roll over to the other side. Do several right and left sets. When this becomes easier, do two complete sets on one side with a brief rest in between before switching sides. When this is no longer difficult, do this same exercise with the leg extended to the front.

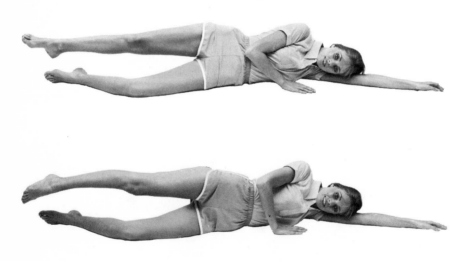

## 4.

### The Bent-Knee Adductor Closing

Lie on your back, bring both knees toward your chest, and then open your legs to the sides, keeping your knees bent. Now, slowly draw your legs together and then slowly lower them back to the open position. Do this five or six times before you rest. Begin with two or three sets, and add more as you grow stronger. Be sure to rest for at least thirty seconds between each set.

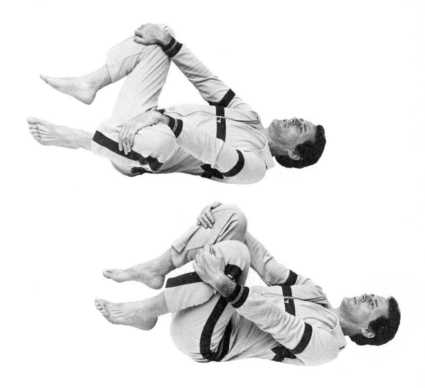

## 5.

### The Sitting Thigh Combination (Out-Up-Down)

While sitting in a chair, first extend one leg out in front of you, parallel to the floor, then bend your knee and lift it as high as you can. Finish by replacing your foot on the floor. Alternate right and left and be sure to keep your back upright. When this becomes easy for you, do three things to increase the demand on your muscles: Raise your knee higher on the lift, extend your foot higher in front of you at the beginning, and repeat the exercise twice in succession before switching legs. Increase slowly over time. Don't overdo it. Keep breathing!

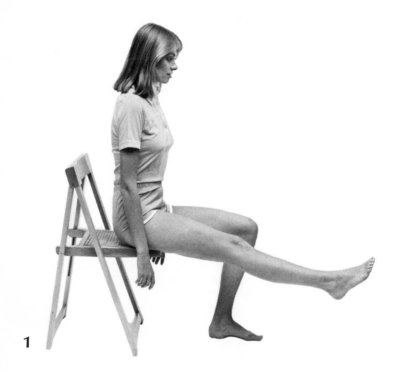

1

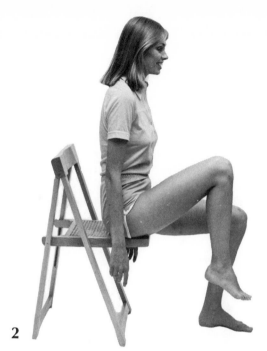

2

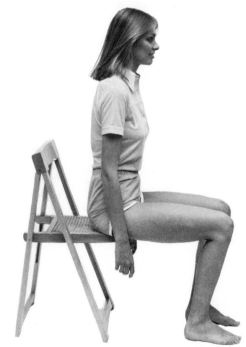

3

## THE ABDOMEN

# 1.

## The Elbow-Knee Touch

Lie on your back and form the shape of an X with your arms and legs. Your feet and your hands should be 3 to 4 feet apart. Touch your left elbow to your right knee. Then return to your original position. Do this without taking your head off the ground, thus keeping neck tension to a minimum. Try to touch your elbow to your knee over the midline of the body, directly above your navel. Alternate sides three or four times and then rest. Begin with two or three sets, slowly increasing their number over time.

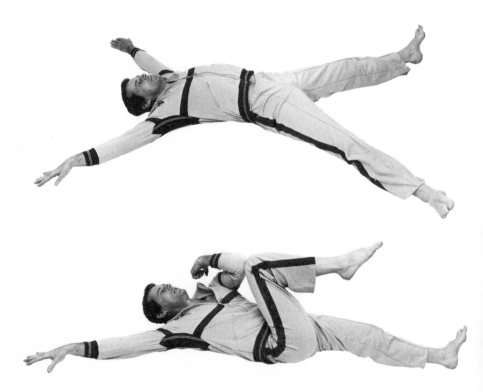

2.

## The Half Abdominal Reach-Across

Lie on your back in the shape of a long X as in the previous exercise. Lift your right hand across your body until you touch the floor at the left side of your waist. Allow your right shoulder and head to rise slightly off the floor as you do this. Then lie back down to your original position. Alternate sides two or three times, rest, and repeat. Increase the number of sets as you get stronger.

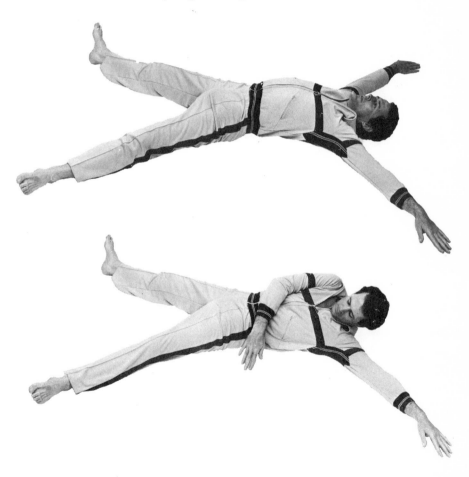

3.

## The Full Abdominal Reach-Across

Stretch out on your back in the same long X position. Now, reach your right hand across your body and touch your left foot. Allow your knees to bend slightly if they want to. As you come up, drag your left hand along the floor, using it for balance and support. Return to the floor rolling down through your back, maintaining the position of your legs. Once again, do two or three right-left alternations. Rest and do a second set. Increase the number of sets over a period of time.

Moving diagonally across the body uses all of the layers of the abdominal muscles. However, only one side of the abdomen is worked at a time, which leaves the other side enough time to recover. Crossing on a diagonal therefore minimizes the strain. For this reason, don't lift straight up as you would in a situp.

If you shake or have to strain, don't continue. Instead, do the Half Abdominal Reach-Across for another week or two.

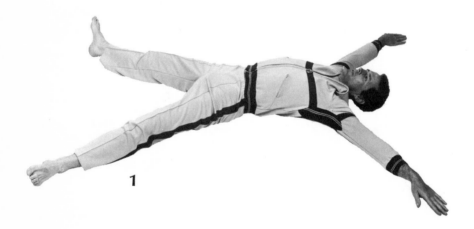

1

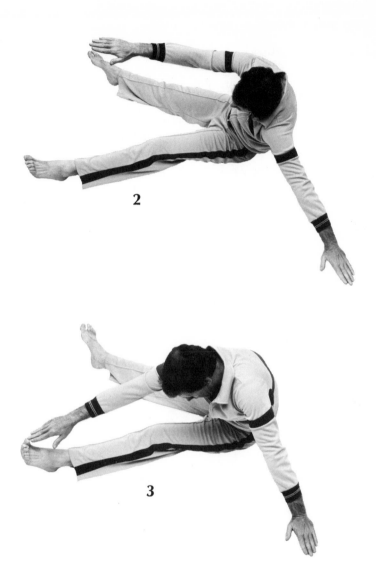

## 4.

## The Pelvic Toss and Roll

Lie on your back with your arms slightly to the side. Lift both knees toward your chest. Without using your arms or lower legs, toss your pelvis up into the air in an arc toward your head. Roll through your back on the way down, keeping your feet in the air.

If you need to push your arms against the floor initially, it's okay. At first, swing your lower legs to help you get the feel of it, but try to eliminate use of your arms and legs as soon as possible. Let your abdominal muscles do the work. Do this movement two or three times. Then rest with your feet on the ground before trying it again.

If you have trouble controlling the downward movement, place a folded towel under the back of your pelvis and make the movement smaller. This will keep you from hitting the ground too hard. If you don't have any control at all, your abdominal muscles are not strong enough for this exercise. Work for a month or two with the Abdominal Reach-Across exercises and the Elbow-Knee Touch to prepare for the Pelvic Toss and Roll.

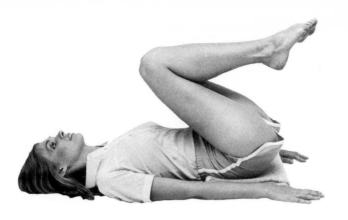

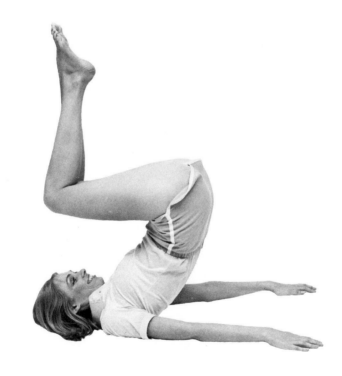

## THE BACK

# 1.

### The Spinal Curve and Reach

Sit on the edge of a chair of the proper height (see page 38) with your feet flat on the floor, parallel and about 12 inches apart. Relax your arms and hands. Shift your weight from side to side in order to feel those two bones in your seat known as the "sit bones." Feel the length of your spine from your sit bones through to the top of your head. While your shoulders remain over your pelvis, slowly curve your spine, allowing your waist to drop back and your head to come forward. Try not to shift your weight forward or backward; simply shrink down. Now, on a slow count of five, begin to unfold from the base of your spine all the way up through the top of your head. When you're as fully upright as possible, without pushing or tightening your muscles, curve the spine once again. Do this three or four times continuously, and then rest. Repeat this sequence three to five times.

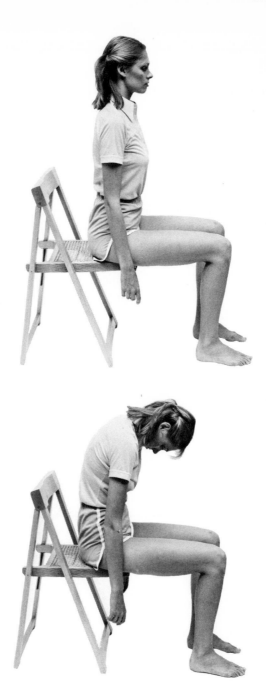

## 2.

## The Back Lift

Sit on the edge of a chair of the proper height with your legs spaced about 2 feet apart. Curve and relax your back and head, while you place your hands on the floor in front of you. From this position you should be able to see through your legs to the wall behind you.

From here, slowly straighten your back without pushing off from the floor with your hands. Inhale as you lift up, and remember that the neck and spine are continuous and should form a fairly straight line. At the end of the upward lift, you should be looking at the floor between your feet, back straight. If possible, observe yourself in a mirror in profile to be sure you're doing this correctly.

Now, slowly round your back and neck forward and return your hands to the floor in the starting position. Exhale as you do this. Rest there for four or five seconds. Repeat the lift three to five times, rest, and then try it again.

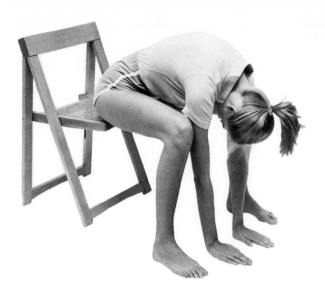

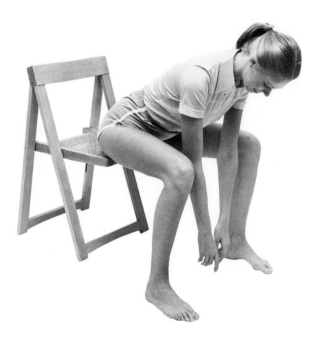

## THE SHOULDERS, ARMS, AND HANDS

# 1.

### The Push-Away*

Stand 2 to 3 feet from a wall. Place your hands on the wall in front of you at shoulder height. Keep your body in a straight line and lean toward the wall. Then push the wall away until you're standing upright again.

Do this five to ten times, rest, and then repeat. As you become more comfortable, place your feet farther out from the wall. Don't move so far away that your heels lift more than a half-inch off the floor. Start with three or four sets and build up to ten.

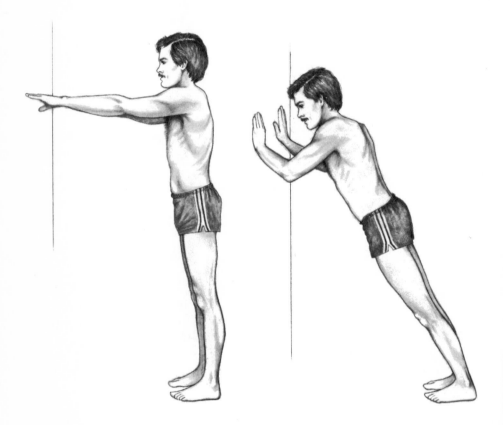

*This is a modification of the push-away exercise in *Total Fitness* by Laurence E. Morehouse and Leonard Gross (New York: Simon and Schuster, 1975), page 187.

## 2.

### Towel-Twisting

Forcefully twist a towel with all your might as if you were wringing it out, as described in the tension-relaxation exercises on page 121. Switch the direction of your hands each time.

## 3.

### Hand Flexion

This exercise has already been described in the section on upper-body warm-ups (see page 91). When you use hand flexion for developing strength in the forearm, do five or six up-and-down sets before switching hands. As you become stronger, progressively increase the number of sets to fifteen to twenty.

## 4.

### The Squeeze

The Squeeze can be done either with a small, flexible ball or with a ball of modeling clay. The exercise is more effective with clay, but many people prefer to use a ball because it's not messy. A "pinky" is probably the best type of ball to use—the one that is rubber all the way through. If you want to use clay and stay clean, try doing it with a small plastic bag on each hand, or put the clay in a plastic bag.

Simply hold the ball or clay in your hand and squeeze it repeatedly. When you become slightly tired, switch to the other hand.

If you are building strength for a specific activity, you shouldn't have to do this exercise for very long. Once you've attained the desired strength, you should be able to maintain it through your sport or exercise program. To keep from getting bored, do the squeeze while you're doing something else, such as watching television or talking on the phone.

# 9

## ALIGNMENT:
## Postural Change
## Through the Use of Imagery

One thing that disturbs optimal functioning and general health is when the body's parts are out of their natural alignment and balance. This is commonly referred to as "bad posture." Most people's idea of posture is static. They picture it as a fixed position, occurring only when one is standing still or sitting down. Posture, or as I prefer to call it, alignment, is with you in every movement. In fact, your alignment when you are moving is just as important as when you are still. The science of the natural alignment of the human skeletal structure and its relationship to injury is a relatively new and unique field.

Most people associate "good posture" with such childhood instructions as "Stand up straight," "Chest out," and "Shoulders back." This tends to fix you into a rigidly held position, which invariably creates increased amounts of tension. The more tension there is, the more uncomfortable you are and the harder it is to move with grace, power, and effectiveness. Consequently, most people abandon their "good posture" for a more comfortable, yet equally destructive slumped and collapsed alignment of their bodies. In good alignment the weight is transferred through your bones with the least amount of stress. You look better and feel better. Optimal alignment is neither rigidly held nor collapsed. On the contrary, it is rather easily movable and gently activated. When you move with good alignment, your body is alive and responsive. Good alignment supports your weight with little effort, as in the resilient readiness of a cat.

*The basic key to optimal alignment is motion.* Keeping things moving and changing even in the smallest ways can help you avoid pain and injury. The body is actually designed to be in motion all the time. Watch someone who is standing "perfectly still" on both feet. If you observe him carefully enough, you'll begin to notice a slight back-and-forth, side-to-side motion. The body naturally sways in a small sideways-figure-8 pattern, because it needs to constantly readjust its balance to keep from toppling over.

Imagine balancing a long, 300-pound steel pole that is standing upright on the ground. It takes very little effort to hold it upright so long as it stays vertically balanced. However, if it begins to tip, you will have to exert tremendous force to keep it from falling, while maintaining it in the tipped position. This is very like the situation in an improperly aligned body. We have to tighten our muscles to hold ourselves up, because our bones are not in an aligned and balanced relationship, and thus we develop excess tension.

When one part of the body is misaligned, it has an adverse effect on the whole system. Such a chain reaction could originate from a birth defect, an old injury that has been compensated for, an emotional problem, or a poor habit learned from an exercise or dance teacher. For example: Limping for a few weeks on a hurt foot causes the injured leg to become weak while the other leg becomes overworked, and over time this can cause tension and pain in the other leg. If your body is out of alignment, you will be very prone to injury. Follow the procedures outlined in this chapter for correcting your alignment and you will be able to exercise more safely. Changing your alignment means replacing the movement patterns and habits that you have maintained for years with new, correct ones. It involves a reeducation of the body and a change of the image that you have of yourself.

## The Use of Imagery

The most effective tool in realigning the body, correcting poor movement habits, and teaching relaxation techniques is the use of Imagery or imagined movement. (A brief history of the development of this revolutionary therapeutic tool is given in the Appendix.) An image is a picture in the mind, a visualization of a thought or feeling or of an experience that is real or imagined. Most people are not aware of how much they use imagery in their lives, or of its basic creative power. We tend to take it for granted, but mental images even affect the way we feel. The mere process of actively imagining and creating a mental picture can be a very effective learning tool.

According to an article in *Research Quarterly*,* an experiment was conducted to determine whether the use of mental images could improve the foul-shooting ability of a group of student basketball players. The test lasted for twenty days, and all the players were scored on the first and last days. One-third of the participants did not practice shooting at all, and they showed no improvement. Another third practiced foul shots every day, and their scores improved by 24 percent. The last group did not engage in physical practice. Instead, they practiced mentally, imagining themselves shooting baskets and correcting their shots if they missed. This group improved 23 percent, practically the same amount as the group that had actually shot baskets every day.

All activity and learning is controlled by the brain. This includes all of our voluntary muscular activities and habits. What occurs when we learn a skill is that we undergo what is called neuromuscular education. A specific nerve pattern is established in the body. The repetition of a particular action ingrains a particular neurologically programmed connection between your brain and different parts of your body. New activities or experiences fall into place just as the flow of water down a mountainside follows the etchings ingrained by previous storms. When we establish a neuromuscular pattern, it becomes deeply embedded and automatic. We usually call this pattern a habit or a skill. Repatterning neurological impulses is what is required to change poor movement habits.

The use of Imagery can change postural alignment. Two approaches can be taken. One involves the very specific images that apply to a particular area or segment of the body, as in "Imagine your spine getting longer," or "Imagine your head floating on top of your spine." The other is the use of more generalized, total-body images which attempt to integrate many of the parts into a unified whole. Different types of images work for different people and for different problems.

---

* Cited in Maxwell Maltz, M.D., *Psycho-Cybernetics* (New York: Pocket Books, 1960), page 35.

Both the texture and quality of an image and the direction of its movement determine its effect on the body, and both must be taken into consideration. For instance, if you imagine your spine as a river flowing upward, out through the top of your head, the net result is one of fluid support and uplift. If you change the direction of the flow and imagine the same river flowing down through your body and out your feet, it results in a sensation of heaviness, compression, and collapse in the spine. Even though the texture of the image remains the same — flowing water — changing the direction from up to down has a counter-productive effect.

Well-meaning but subtly negative images and ideas often ingrain poor movement habits which are difficult to break. Such counter-productive images as those invoked by the familiar "Keep your chin in," "Hold your head back," "Keep your spine straight," "Lift up," "Shoulders back," and "Breathe abdominally" actually result in excess muscle tension and forced postural alignment, paving the way for injury.

Try this: *Imagine your head is as buoyant as a balloon filled with helium, with your spine flowing upward like a river. Feel your legs and feet as feather-light with liquid joints. Now glide across the floor, as if you were walking on air.*

As a teacher at American University in Washington, D.C., Carol Boggs developed new uses of Imagery in work with postural realignment and movement habits. She headed a team that developed an approach to movement problems called Dynamic Alignment. She created a construct which identified four broad categories to describe people's general movement habits: *collapse, rigid, overkill,* and *ac-tivate.* These categories are helpful in understanding how our ideas about movement affect the way we move and in teaching good body alignment.

When told to relax, most people think *"collapse,"* or "slump down." They feel sluggish or heavy and drop their weight, putting stress on the joints of the spine and legs. The body should feel buoyant, and not dropped. The image of relaxing up instead of (collapsing) down can improve your alignment and help you move more easily.

People who are *rigid* in their movement move as if against a con-stant resistance. It looks as if they are holding back. Their movements are stiff and often awkward. People who are rigid have a limited movement range and tire easily because they are always moving against their own tension. They usually end up building more tension.

*Overkill* describes the general movement patterns of the person who is hard to take, works too hard, always uses too much force, and builds up a sweat in the simplest of activities. He believes that if it doesn't hurt it won't do any good.

The collapse, rigid, and overkill approaches to movement waste energy and work against your optimal movement potential.

The concept of *activation* creates an easy-going, alive involvement in moving. When you are activated, you move your body efficiently and economically, using the appropriate amount of effort—not more, not less. Your movements are full and free. As you sit or stand, there is a feeling of "upness," without tension. When you move, you have a floating, buoyant feeling.

You see these concepts expressed every day in the way different people shake your hand. A collapsed handshake will feel like a limp dishrag or a dead fish. A rigid handshake will feel tense and resistant. An overkill handshake feels like it will break your hand. An activated handshake will feel warm and firm, yet gentle.

In order for a movement pattern to change, something has to happen in the brain and in the thought process itself. When you use Imagery, you don't try to *do* anything. Actively trying to change doesn't work with this method. Repatterning involuntary nerve responses is best done through visualization, or allowing a movement to happen as a result of directive thought.

## SOLVING ALIGNMENT PROBLEMS

There are several professionally developed approaches to alignment problems that share a movement perspective and a reliance on various Imagery techniques. These include the Alexander Technique, the Bartinieff Fundamentals as part of Effort/Shape Analysis, Ideo-Kinetic Facilitation, and Muscular Therapy. For more information on these approaches, see the Appendix. Effecting a permanent change in postural alignment is not an easy task. It takes a good eye, in-depth training, and years of experience. From my experience, professionals trained in the above approaches are very effective in helping people learn new patterns of improved alignment. However, there is much that motivated individuals can do to improve their alignment on their own.

What follows is an analysis of the key areas of the body that are essential for good body alignment. For convenience, they are arranged from the ankle to the head. Each section is followed by specific exercises and Imagery techniques designed to improve alignment, some of which integrate several parts of the body.

## THE ANKLES

A joint is the place where two bones meet. Each joint is built to move in a particular way. Movement of the body through space always occurs by the contraction of a muscle that crosses at least one joint. A muscle contracts by shortening and pulls the bones into a new position, producing movement. That's how it works.

When bones only move through one plane, as in a forward-and-back direction, we call the joint a hinge joint. The ankle is a hinge joint designed to move forward and back, but it also has a certain degree of side-to-side mobility. This extra mobility is necessary for walking on uneven surfaces, which is the way the world was before concrete sidewalks. Without this maneuverability at the ankle, we would constantly lose our balance, fall down, and probably break our legs. Even though such sports as basketball and tennis are played on flat surfaces, full mobility of the ankle is necessary for quick side-to-side or turning movements.

Structurally, the ankle is very vulnerable to injury, especially at the outer side of the joint. Unfortunately, many people develop the habit of walking with their feet pointing slightly outward, or sometimes inward, rather than straight ahead and parallel to each other. Small deviations of outward or inward rotation of the foot within an inch are often of minor consequence, but absolute parallel is best. This ensures an all-around development of strength in the muscles that support the ankle and lower leg.

There are several ways in which the structure of the ankle can be disturbed. A primary cause of ankle disturbance is fallen arches. If you have congenital flat feet, you were born with a flat arch and there's nothing you can do about it. You have developed strength in this position since childhood and for the most part you can function well.

If you have a functionally fallen or dropped arch, it is probably caused by poor ankle-knee alignment and can be changed with corrective work. Sometimes the source of the alignment problem is an imbalance in the mechanical structure of the foot. Such an imbalance can be corrected only with a balanced, molded arch support called an "orthotic." Ideally, when you walk with your feet and knees pointed

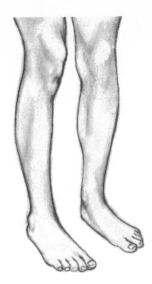

straight ahead of you in a parallel position, your arch should give a little when you step on it and then spring back to normal with each step.
When the arch is in a constantly dropped position, the knee is usually
turned inward in relation to the foot. A functionally dropped arch
often begins because the knee is chronically turned in.

The ankle is "at the bottom of the pile"—more weight passes
through it than through any other single joint. The ankle is totally
dependent on alignment for its health. Deviations from the parallel
position here often cause problems in other parts of the body. The
arch, the ankle, the knee, and the hip have an intricate movement
relationship. When one goes out of line, the others generally follow.
When working with your ankle alignment, bear in mind that the for-
ward-to-back movement is primary and the side-to-side movement
secondary. Try to maintain a proper alignment by walking, running,
and standing with your feet in a parallel position.

To change poor ankle alignment in the most efficient way, you must
first reduce the tension in the foot and leg. Then work on moving in
this new alignment, which will in turn condition and strengthen your
foot and leg muscles.

*Exercise 1 is a preparatory exercise to increase mobility before
working on the alignment.*

# 1.

## Knee Shakes

Sit on the edge of a chair of the proper height (see page 38) with your feet parallel, about 12 inches apart. Loosely move your knees together and apart. Don't be concerned if your feet don't remain completely on the floor. Now, continue with one leg at a time and try to keep the bottom of your foot flat on the floor. You will notice that either the outside or inside of each foot characteristically comes off the floor. That is the place you'll have to watch.

Next, shake both knees together, trying to keep the soles of both feet flat on the floor. Follow this by standing up with your feet parallel, about 12 inches apart, knees slightly bent. Move your knees rather quickly apart and together as you did in the sitting position, while maintaining a parallel position with your feet flat on the floor.

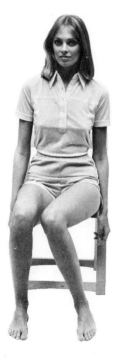
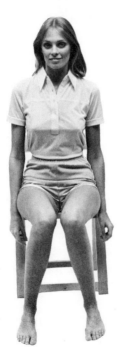
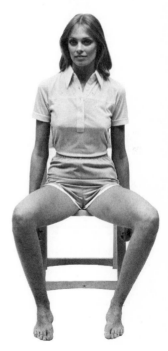

## 2.

### The Elbow-Knee Lean

This exercise is described in the strength-building exercises on page 164. Here we are not so much concerned with how heavily you lean onto your leg, but with lining up the knee directly over the foot.

## 3.

### The Two-Legged Stance

Over the next day or so, while you stand, try to become conscious of your postural habits. See if you stand on one leg or both, and if your feet are parallel, turned out, or turned in. If you want to change a long-ingrained habit, first you must become aware of it and then try to change it whenever you notice it. Whenever you think of it, try to stand on both feet equally, with your feet parallel and about shoulder width apart. Do this at the elevator, or on line at the grocer, the bus, or the bank. Don't lock your knees. Keep them slightly slack and ready so that you can move easily in any direction at any time.

## 4.

### Parallel Walking

If you constantly walk with your feet turned out and your knees pointed straight ahead, you are reinforcing poor alignment. Try walking looking down at your feet for at least five minutes once or twice a day. At other times glance down occasionally to check if you're walking parallel. Get to know the body feeling of walking parallel so that you won't always have to look.

Try this image in your parallel walking. *Imagine that you are walking on a very narrow railroad track the width of your stance. As you walk, keep your feet on the tracks.*

If it's too difficult to do parallel walking or if it hurts your feet or knees, you haven't progressed far enough with your other exercises yet, so wait awhile.

## THE KNEES

The knee is a hinge joint, with practically no side-to-side movement. It is extremely vulnerable to poor alignment. In many cases the alignment of the knee depends upon that of the foot and ankle and also the hip. For example, if the knee moves straight ahead and the foot turns outward when you walk, a twist or torque occurs at the knee joint. This is the key knee-alignment problem that causes the most serious leg injuries in sports and exercise. It is also the least understood. When people with this knee problem stand with their feet parallel, they feel "pigeon-toed." This is because habit has locked the foot and leg muscles into an improper relationship, and so standing with the feet parallel in turn makes their knees face inward toward each other. In order to walk with their knees moving straight forward, they turn their feet outward. This stance is a compensation for poor lower-leg alignment that has become muscularly set and rigid. The problem can originate either in the foot or the knee. There is usually tension at the inner part of the lower leg and weakness at the outer portion. The inner section of the knee joint must continually absorb abnormal amounts of stress if you walk and move this way.

Infants's feet are often turned in. This is quite normal, and nothing to worry about. A young child's lower leg rotates outward to the straight position usually by age 2 or 2½. Pigeon-toedness in an older child or an adult can result from the lower leg's not rotating as it should. Another cause is excess muscular tension in the inner thigh and inward rotator muscles. Being toed-in is less frequent and does not cause as many injuries as being toed-out.

Another alignment problem at the knee joint is the so-called hyperextended knee. In this case, the knees pass through the functionally straight position in standing and bend backward. This places stress on the knee joint, its cartilage and ligaments, the ankle joint, and all the muscles of the lower leg and thigh. It throws the weight of the body off-center and backward onto the heels. This causes the muscles to work incorrectly in order to compensate. Hyperextended knees can be especially dangerous in sports, exercise, and particularly dancing, contributing to knee injuries, calf spasms, torn muscles, and sprained ankles.

Accidents involving the knee do not always happen by accident. There is often a preexisting vulnerability due to poor alignment which

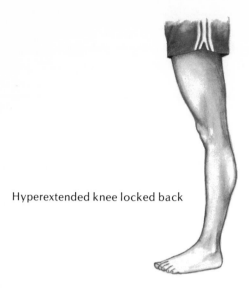

Hyperextended knee locked back

makes us susceptible to injury. Basketball players don't have weak legs, but they often have extremely poor knee alignment, which puts their legs under enormous physical stress. It is no wonder that professional basketball players and athletes suffer so many knee injuries.

In fifteen years of therapeutic work with people, I have found that the overwhelming majority of knee problems originate from poor alignment and its resultant constant tension. To check your knee alignment, first stand with your feet in parallel position. Bend your knees as you normally would, trying to keep your back upright and your heels and all five toes on the floor. (Refer to the photo.) As you look down at your feet, you should see your inner arch and two to two-and-a-half toes on the inner side of each foot. If you can't, your knees are turned in.

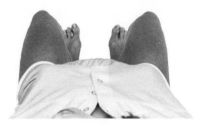

If you can gently and easily move your knees apart and see your toes without pushing, you will have an easier time correcting your alignment. It means that you have some flexibility but uneven muscle development and no strength in the well-aligned position. If you cannot keep your feet parallel without discomfort, or if you have trouble opening your knees, your misalignment is very bound and set muscularly. The muscles will have to be relaxed first, stretched second, and then realigned. You can't sculpt rock-hard clay; you have to soften it first.

# 1.

## Parallel Knee Bends

This is a very basic exercise, used for many purposes. You've seen it in your fitness test and as part of the lower-body warm-up. Here we will add a few things to it.

Stand with your feet parallel, about 4 to 6 inches apart. Simply bend your knees as far as you can, keeping your back upright and your heels on the ground. There are three things to concentrate on. First, your knees should go directly over the center of your feet. You can try to do this in two ways. Imagine the center of your knee going directly over your second toe. Or look down, keeping your back upright, and see if you can see two to three toes on the inside of each foot as shown in the photo opposite. This means you are sending your knees directly over your toes in good alignment. Second, be aware of the three joints involved in a Knee Bend. Imagine your three joints folding—the ankle, the knee, and particularly the hip. Each time you bend, imagine that you are going to sit. Third, think of sending your knees forward, not down. A good way to do this exercise is facing a mirror so you can see what is happening more easily.

Do these Knee Bends slowly, six to eight at a time, followed by a break. Concentrate on one aspect at a time and then try to put them together.

## 2.

## Foot-Knee Flexion

Lie on your back and raise one leg in the air with your knee bent at about a 90-degree angle and your foot flexed. Look over the top of your knee and line up your foot and knee so that the front of your foot is centered and frames your knee (see diagram).

When the alignment is correct, begin to point and flex your foot so that your foot returns to this framed position with each flexion. If your knees are chronically turned in when you flex your foot, most of your foot will tend to appear on the outside of the knee.

Do six to eight flexions before changing legs. After this becomes easy, try straightening your knee each time you point your foot. Move your foot diagonally out from the body (not straight up toward the ceiling). See if you can return to the framed position directly, without making adjustments. After you get the hang of this, try it with your eyes closed, only opening them to check your position at the end of each flexion.

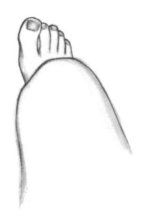

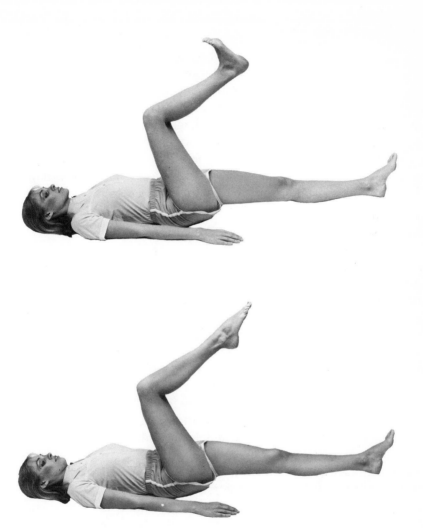

3.

## The Slacked-Knee Stance

This one is good for people who have hyperextended knees and those who stand with their knees locked. It is, simply, to always have your knees slacked or very slightly bent. You can think about this on line at the bank along with your parallel-foot position. Try to catch yourself whenever your knees lock back. Put little signs up in your bathroom, your kitchen, and your office that say, "Jane—knees," "Henry—knees easy," or "Sonja—don't lock." They may seem silly as you write them, but they are helpful. Never leave the same sign up for more than a week or two or you won't notice it anymore.

## THE LOWER BACK, ABDOMEN, AND PELVIS

It is impossible to speak of the alignment of the pelvis, lower back, and abdominal areas separately. They are as interdependent as the neck and head. When one moves, the other must follow like the two sides of a coin.

Within this area of the body people are often quite preoccupied with their protuding middles and buttocks. Many strive to tuck them in to get them out of the way. This can create undue stress and lead to many problems. Sucking your belly in to get rid of your fat is like sweeping the dirt under the rug—it's still there. If it's fat that you have hanging out in front, losing weight is the way to change the problem. But, more often than not, the extremely protruding middle is caused by poor lower-back and pelvic alignment and not by fat at all. When the natural forward curve of the lower spine is accentuated and increased, intense pressure is built up at the apex of that forward curve, which is at the lower back. The most dangerous part of this common "swayback" posture is that unnatural stress is placed on the lower-back muscles, the vertebrae, and the discs.

When standing in correct alignment, the bones of the pelvis are straight up and down rather than tilted forward or back, the buttock muscles produce a natural curve to the back, and there is a slight forward curve in the lower back. The abdomen also naturally curves slightly outward in the front. Soft and supple bellies are a lot healthier than tight, rock-hard ones. That's not to say that the muscles of the abdomen should not be strong. When there is good alignment, the muscles of the abdomen and lower back are activated and used for balance, not for holding you in a rigid, upright position. Most people have difficulty accepting the idea of a soft belly and a relaxed pelvis, let alone considering it desirable.

If you are standing in good alignment, the superficial muscles of the lower back and abdomen are fairly relaxed. The greatest amount of work should be done by the psoas muscles, which run diagonally through your lower body from the top of your lower back through your pelvis, attaching to the upper, inner part of the thighs. These muscles are very deep and can barely be felt by hand pressure. They are the most important postural muscles.

Put the book down and stand up for a minute. Now, place your fingers on your lower-back muscles, one on each side. Hyperextend your pelvis by making your buttocks stick out in back, let your abdomen fall forward, and feel how tense the lower-back muscles become. Now, while remaining in that position, very gently bounce up and down on your heels with straight knees. You will feel the jarring effect in your lower back. The shock of impact is being absorbed there. Relax now.

This is what happens when you stand and move with the pelvis out of alignment. With every jump, with every jog, with every step, the lower back is jarred and brutalized. We do this even when we fall into a chair, and plop ourselves down. It's no wonder that in 1977 seventy million visits to doctors were made because of back pain and twenty million of those were for chronic low-back pain.

Muscular strength is only a minor factor in alignment. There are many misconceptions about strength as it relates to posture and particularly to the pelvis and lower back. People who have very strong backs and abdominal muscles frequently have poor postural alignment and people with relatively weaker muscles often have excellent postural alignment.

Poor alignment of the lower back and pelvis creates deep tension that can lead to severe pain and spasm. In order for you to attain good alignment, it is essential that the lower-back, buttock, and abdominal muscles be capable of relaxing. Enough tension must be removed so that forceful pressure on the back muscles does not cause pain; then realignment work should begin. This is best accomplished by the type of alignment exercises that follow, which strive to alter neuromuscular habit patterns through the use of imagery.

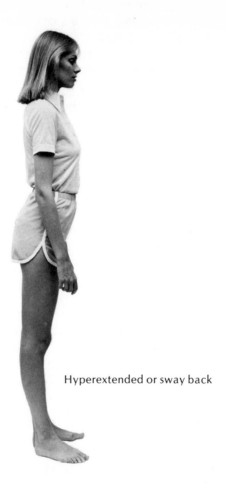

Hyperextended or sway back

Correct placement of the pelvis is dependent on its relationship to the thigh and the lower back. Keep them all in mind as you work with alignment here. To begin, try Exercises 1 and 2 to increase mobility first, before working with the alignment directly in Exercises 3 and 4. The ability to perform the Pelvic Swing without forcefully tightening the abdominal or lower-back muscles is one of the first prerequisites to working toward better alignment of the torso.

# 1.

## The Pelvic Tilt and Lift

This exercise is detailed on page 58 of the general body warm-ups.

# 2.

## The Pelvic Swing

In a slight Parallel Knee Bend, gently swing your pelvis forward and back with minimal tension in the lower back and abdomen. (The Pelvic Swing is described fully in the tension chapter on page 123.)

*This begins our direct alignment work.*

# 3.

## Parallel Knee Bends from the Sacrum

As you do the Parallel Knee Bends, have your weight on the whole foot, send your knees forward, and really try to feel the fold in the hip joint, as described previously in the section on knee alignment (see page 195. As you bend, imagine a plumb line with a weight attached to it hanging from the end of your tailbone, toward the floor. When you straighten, keep moving upward, lengthening your legs, and continue imagining the weight of the plumb line pulling downward. Don't let your knees go back into a locked or hyperextended position at all; this will cause the pelvis to tip.

# 4.

## Headlight Walking

Feel where the fronts of your hip bones are with your hands and *imagine there is a headlight mounted on each bone. As you walk, envision them shining straight in front of you.* If they shine on the floor, your pelvis is hyperextended. If they shine upward, the pelvis is tucked under. When the pelvis is erect, they shine straight ahead. Walk around using this image for ten minutes twice a day.

## THE CHEST

The chest or rib-cage area includes the center back, upper back, and shoulder blades. The natural range of movement in this area is rather small. Rotation and side-bending are inhibited by the ribs, which are fixed into the spine. Bending backward is also limited by the structure of the vertebrae in that area.

In good alignment, the chest is balanced over the pelvis. When it is out of line, it is usually either too far forward or too far back. In scoliosis, it is pushed to the side.

A very common alignment problem in this area is the "collapsed chest," which generally brings the shoulders rounding forward. To balance the weight, the neck juts slightly forward and the lower-back curve increases, tipping the bottom of the pelvis backward. This places

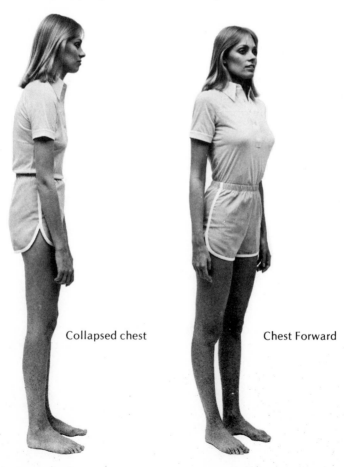

Collapsed chest                    Chest Forward

extra weight and pressure on the lower back. (This position of the pelvis is often referred to as swayback.) With the thousands of people I have worked with, it has been my experience that these combined problems make up the most prevalent postural-alignment problem in our society.

Besides being collapsed or back, the chest is also often held high or puffed up, like Bruno's in the *Popeye* cartoons. This is referred to as the chronic inspiratory position. Inhale deeply for a moment in your upper chest. Now exhale, keeping your chest in that high position. Do this several times and you will begin to experience tension and pain somewhere between your shoulders or in your chest. Many people suffer with this continually as a part of their alignment-tension syndrome. It gets its fancy name — chronic inspiratory — because people

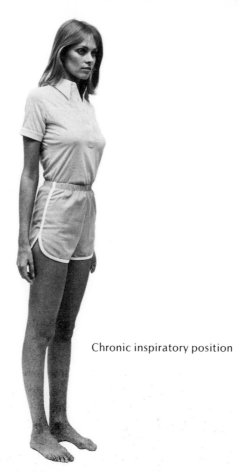

Chronic inspiratory position

look like they're holding their inhaled position all the time. This posture severely limits your breathing capacity, because you never exhale fully. The exhale is the most important and difficult aspect of breathing. If it is not complete, the muscles of the chest never get a chance to relax. Furthermore, there is always a certain amount of carbon dioxide which remains stagnant in your lungs, setting a fixed limitation on the amount of fresh air and oxygen you can take in. When you don't completely exhale, you maintain what's referred to as a residual volume of air in your lungs.

Many chest-alignment problems have to do with breathing disturbances often caused by emotional difficulties, not the mechanical kind of difficulties I have been describing. This makes the chest an area that must be approached with great care and sensitivity so as not to interfere with the established emotional equilibrium.

*If your chest is collapsed, do loosening Exercises 1 and 2 for a while in preparation for working on the alignment.*

# 1.

## The Large-Ball Chest Release

See page 122 for the details of this technique.

# 2.

## The Chest Reach (Forward and Back)

Sit upright on a chair of the proper height (see page 38), feet flat on the floor, parallel, and about 12 inches apart. Slowly reach forward with your chest as far as you can and then reach back with your chest into a rounded position. First try breathing in on the forward movement and out as you go back. Then try breathing out when you go forward and in as you go back. After it's easy to do the Chest Reach sitting, try it standing with your knees slightly bent.

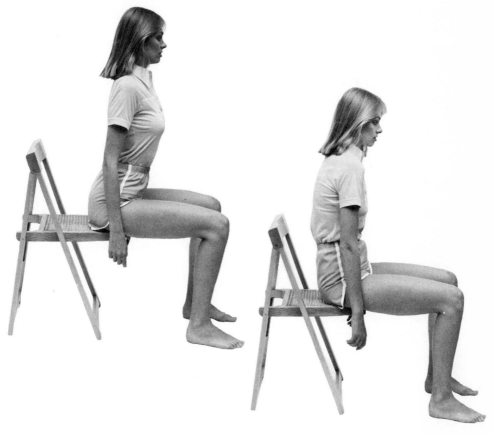

## 3.

### The Spinal Curve and Reach

This exercise, described on page 178 of the strength chapter, is also good for working on alignment. Concentrate on the sequential lengthening of the spine, imagining that the movement begins at the tailbone. When you've reached the full upright position, check to make sure that your shoulders are relaxed, you are looking straight forward, and your head is easily balanced, hovering on the top of your spine.

## 4.

### Image Walking

Now try a few Imagery exercises to unify your approach and involve more of your mind and whole body. As you walk, *imagine a gently strong breeze blowing upward from the center of your pelvis through your chest and out the top of your head.* Try to do this for at least three or four minutes at a time. Here is another one to try. *Imagine that there is a magnet above your head, drawing you toward the sky as you walk.* Don't try to do anything. Just picture this in your mind and see what happens.

## 5.

### The River Walk

*Imagine there is an upward-flowing river inside your body, constantly pouring out the top of your head like a fountain. See the water fall down along the outside of your body.* This image enables you to support the upwardness of your body from its center while maintaining a softness and a relaxed quality in your arms, shoulders, and rib cage.

## THE SHOULDERS

The shoulder area includes the two bones which make up the shoulder girdle—the scapula, or shoulder blade, and the clavicle, or collarbone—plus the upper arm as part of the shoulder joint and the upper back. It is impossible to consider these body parts separately because they always work together, one affecting the other.

When the shoulder is properly aligned, there is a balance between the musculature of the chest, shoulder, and upper back, allowing the scapula to lie flat on the back of the rib cage. The inner border of the scapula is then almost parallel to the spine. The shoulder blades cannot be forced into position or held in position without inducing a lot of tension. In good shoulder alignment, there is a feeling of length between the neck and the shoulders, as well as a feeling of width across the chest and upper back.

Misalignment of the shoulders is intimately connected with the problems of shoulder tension, muscle weakness, and negative alignment habits resulting in a collapsed chest and spine. These sometimes result from poor exercise or dance training. Tension is clearly involved when the shoulders are constantly raised. When the shoulders are pulled back, tension and training are the likely causes. If the shoulders are rotated forward, with the shoulder blades sticking out in the back and the chest collapsed, a combination of factors is at work. Other shoulder postures that are often seen include: the shoulders pulled back and down sharply in a military stance, the shoulder blades pinched together, and one shoulder higher than the other. The latter is often caused by a spinal deviation, as in cases of scoliosis, a sideways curve of the spine.

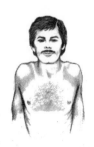

Constantly raised

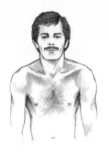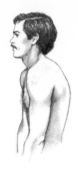

Rotated forward

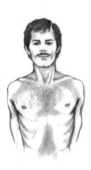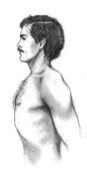

Military stance

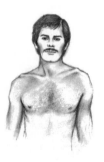

One shoulder higher

Shoulder problems can also be caused by certain occupations. If you crane over a desk or drawing board eight hours a day, work in a hunched position (as a welder does, for instance), or drive a truck or car for a living, you may develop poor shoulder alignment.

Poor alignment here is inseparably related to the placement of the chest, upper back, head, and neck. So, do the alignment exercises for those areas and at the same time imagine that your arms are bone earrings hanging off your spine. You shouldn't have to hold your shoulders in place. They should just hang there.

Poor shoulder alignment is also often caused by excess muscle tension. If this is the case, try some of the tension-release exercises and ball techniques for the whole upper body described in the tension chapter.

## THE HEAD AND NECK

Head and neck alignment are inseparably related. When you stand properly, the back of your neck should have a natural slight forward curve; it was not built to be straight up and down. Your head should balance gently at the top of your spine, and the muscles surrounding the neck should only have to work minimally. In balancing the head in this way, the neck muscles remain relatively soft to the touch. If you place your hand on the back of your neck and project your head several inches forward, you'll feel the muscles of the neck contract. Even if you hold your neck as little as an inch out of line, there is a constant buildup of neck tension. The head is generally the heaviest single part of the body and weighs anywhere from 10 to 15 pounds. If

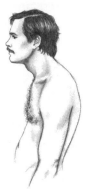

Head and neck projected forward

you imagine holding a 15-pound weight by your teeth for a few minutes, you will begin to get an idea of how much tension is built when you hold your head forward and out of line. Your muscles have to hold your head up instead of balancing it. The forward projection of the head and neck is the most common neck-alignment problem that there is.

When the head is out of line, it is often tilted slightly to one side. There can also be a combination of head projected forward and head slightly tilted. If the head is tilted, there is continual stress on the muscles of the side you are tilted toward. People with this problem commonly have trouble lying prone with their head to one side. They may have a tendency to get stiff necks, one-sided neck spasms, or pinched nerves in the neck.

Sometimes the head is tilted toward the back with the chin raised. This places stress on the muscles of the occiput, in back of your neck just below the skull. You have probably experienced stiffness and tension there if you've ever sat too close to the screen at the movies or sat at a bar and watched a television high up near the ceiling. If you try tilting your head back 2 inches and hold it there for a full two or three minutes, you will begin to feel tension or pain creep into the upper part of the back of your neck. This posture often goes along with chronically raised shoulders.

When correcting head and neck alignment, it should first be determined whether or not the neck muscles can relax enough to adjust easily to the new alignment. Second, the neck muscles should be flexible enough to move into this new alignment. If the muscles of the neck are either extremely tense or inflexible, I have found that they respond to change faster if they are softened first, and then made flexible through various neck-stretching exercises. Finally, with the use of Imagery and guided movement, you experience a new way of balancing your head on top of your spine. With time and guidance you can learn how to integrate this into your movement habits.

In working with head and neck alignment, it is important to realize that the head is a separate entity from the neck. Most people tend to freeze that connection in a forward position. This reduces the blood supply to the brain and often constricts the throat and vocal chords.

The discovery of the importance of head and neck alignment in movement was made by F. M. Alexander, the originator of the Alexander Technique (see the Appendix). Many others have adapted or been influenced by his discoveries, including myself.

# 1.

## The Head Push

Project your head forward and backward as far as you can in both directions without straining, like a chicken moving its head and neck. Relax your mouth and breathe. Do this five to ten times, whenever you feel tight. This exercise is fully detailed in the tension chapter, page 119.

# 2.

## Yes and No

So that you know exactly where the head and neck connect, place one finger in each ear and nod your head in a yes motion. Imagine that your fingers form the axis for your head's movement. Now remove your fingers. On this axis is the top of your neck. In a sitting position, begin to move your head continuously in a yes motion with very small movements. Imagine that your head rotates around this axis. After you have done this for a while, do the same thing saying no with easy small movements. It is important that the yes and no movements be kept very small, barely perceivable. This helps to keep the movement happening high at the top of the spine, where most of us tend to hold a fixed position. Now, try it standing up and then walking slowly. Do this for five to ten minutes daily for about a week just sitting and walking. When you can do this quite easily, try it while doing various activities such as picking things up, writing, typing, driving in traffic, and the like. After a good deal of work at this, try saying yes and no simultaneously. Your head will gently hover at the top of your spine making irregular circular movements. Try this sitting first and then progress slowly to doing it while engaging in some normal activities.

# 10

# KNOW YOUR SPORT
# OR EXERCISE ACTIVITY

"Know thyself" are fine words of advice. This is as true when it comes to exercise and sports as it is for life in general. In order to exercise safely and without pain, you have to know where you are vulnerable to injury, and the limits of your strength. This understanding then allows you to develop the right warm-up and strengthening program for yourself. Each of us should have a tailor-made exercise program designed to meet his or her individual needs. The tests, examples, exercises, and general information included in this book make it possible to avoid pain and the fear of injury while staying physically fit. So take the time to formulate a program to prepare you for your sport. The additional information in this chapter, about preparing yourself for specific sports, which are listed in alphabetical order, will help you to design the best possible personal warm-up and exercise system for the sport you like to play.

## BADMINTON

Badminton can be a tremendously strenuous sport, especially if you are playing singles. Always warm up, paying special attention to your arms, legs, and wrists. Since badminton is usually played on lawns with uneven surfaces, sprained ankles are the most common injury. Be sure to remove any rocks and fill any holes that may exist. Check the area periodically for such danger spots—especially after bad weather, or if you have a dog who likes to bury bones.

## BASEBALL AND SOFTBALL

Baseball and softball are upper-and lower-body sports, so a thorough warm-up is essential.

A major problem in baseball and softball is that you do a lot of standing around and sitting, waiting for something to happen, often for five or ten minutes or more at a time. Keeping warm is the main task. Infielders are better off, because they are usually moving a fair amount of time. If you play outfield, especially left field, you need to keep your body moving. I suggest moving your shoulders up and down and in circles, and frequently doing several side steps to your right and then to your left, almost as if you were fencing or shadowboxing. Punching your hand into the mitt and circling your arm are also good.

Baseball and softball are also tense games. Excitement and anxiety build and there isn't enough activity to discharge the tension, especially when your team is up at bat. Taking a rest when you come in from the field is fine, but three or four minutes before it's your turn at bat, begin to repeat some of your warm-up exercises before or instead of going into the hole to swing the bat. Do a few for the lower body and a few for the arms and shoulders. Get your heart rate and your breathing elevated before you get up to the plate.

Taking good care of your arm is especially important. This is where most ballplayers get hurt. Arm problems frequently occur when you try throwing too far or too hard before you're ready. After your general and upper/lower-body combination warm-ups, begin to throw easily, at about 20 yards, increasing in speed and distance over a ten-or fifteen-minute period. Try to catch the ball in the right place—in the pocket—to avoid catching injuries to the hand or fingers. Reach up to meet the ball, then allow your hand to move back with it, so that your palm or fingers don't have to absorb the impact.

Many injuries occur in amateur softball and baseball and on some professional teams because a player is hesitant to slide or doesn't know how to slide properly. If you hesitate, you will almost certainly be injured. Learn how to slide correctly so that this fear can be overcome. Before the season, players should practice daily until they are expert and confident. Even after the season starts, practice sliding once or twice a week. Ankle sprains and breaks and a variety of knee injuries occur when a metal spike gets hooked into the ground or the base, or when a straight leg slams into the base and doesn't bend to absorb the impact.

There are five or six different types of slides. The head-first slide is the most dangerous because of head and hand injuries and many coaches discourage it, especially when steel cleats are in use. The largest number of injuries occur with the bent-leg slide. You should learn your slides on both sides equally, because if you are forced into a slide on an unfamiliar side you are more likely to hurt yourself. There are two ways to do a bent-leg slide. The safer is to hold your top leg in the air, bringing the leg down onto the base when it is above it. The more experienced slider can extend the leg (don't lock the knee) into the front part of the base. The trouble starts when you decide to slide too late and hit the base too soon with your knee locked. When learning how to slide, always begin on wet grass. Practice barefoot or in tennis shoes. In the junior leagues, before high school, it is usually wise to use the molded-cleat shoe and not steel cleats, because it is safer. The best time to learn how to slide is in the little leagues, between the ages of 8 and 12, when fear is at a minimum and our bodies are most agile.

Whatever your favorite slide is, be good at it. As soon as you touch the base, bend your knee. Keep your leg extended, but never locked.

Catchers often end up with knee problems caused by sitting into the knee joint for extended periods of time. Tension around the knee and a lack of movement cause the synovial fluid in the joint to partially dry up, making the knee incapable of sustaining sudden, quick movements that come in spurts without ill effect. When your legs are cold, the knees absorb the force. I recommend that catchers stand up after every other throw and frequently stand on their knees, using knee pads, during practice.


## BASKETBALL

Basketball is one of the most strenuous and demanding of all sports. It combines almost all aspects of physical fitness. The most common injuries in basketball are those to the lower body. Ankle sprains and strains, adductor and front-thigh strains, hamstring pulls, and Achilles tendinitis start the long list of basketball injuries. Outer-ankle sprains may be slightly more common than knee problems, but knee injuries are more serious. Knee problems occur for a variety of reasons: lack of proper warm-up, poor alignment, excess tension in the legs, and poor surfaces. Unfortunately, young people often play on concrete schoolyard surfaces, constantly jamming the bones of the knee and ankle. After ten years of such wear and tear on the knee, it is no wonder that so many professional basketball players suffer severe and debilitating knee injuries which often end their careers. In addition, basketball players are subject to frequent shin splints. They can be a serious problem in themselves but are often the forerunner of more serious injury.

Accumulated muscle tension and chronic muscle spasms are also an important factor in many basketball injuries. In basketball you must be strong, but loose. Tension inhibits the basketball player and makes him more prone to the above-listed injuries. Back spasms and hamstring pulls are more likely to occur where there is excess tension buildup.

Professional basketball players are usually nursing along at least one injury after the first month or two of the season. They understand that warm-up and flexibility are important, but many go about it in an inefficient manner. The amateur, the weekend basketball player or the winter basketball enthusiast is often badly injured because he is not in condition on a year-round basis. To plunge into a sport like basketball without a month of preparation can be very dangerous physically. Always warm up thoroughly before playing basketball.

If you plan to play basketball for the first time, or if you have not played for a long time, prepare yourself gradually. Start by running to build strength and endurance. Next do some jumping, first jumping rope and then higher jumps, making sure that your alignment is correct and that your heels make contact before takeoff and upon landing. Then begin to run figure-8s and to do start-and-stop running for increasing periods of time. Start playing the game easily and with reserve for a few weeks before you let go into it. The key word is moderation—move into it slowly. For the amateur, as well as the professional, alignment in movement is one of the most important aspects of basketball, and is perhaps the least known. It accounts for more injuries than would be suspected, and many of these could be avoided if work in this area were included in training.

## BICYCLING

The most common noncollision injuries in bicycling are outer-calf pain, knee pain, and chronic soreness of the hands. In this sport, your overall safety depends on good equipment. Always buy a good-quality bike, which will stay finely tuned. It may need adjustment, but not unreasonably often. Inexpensive bikes, especially the 10-speed variety, can go out of adjustment within a few weeks. You will need to tune your bike every two to three months, and it may need an oiling even if you have not ridden it.

Men's bikes are structurally sounder than women's bikes and are being used increasingly by women. Lights in the front and back of the bike are essential, as are pants clips or rubber bands to prevent your pants from catching in the chain. In addition, during night riding you should always dress so that you can be seen, and a red leg light is safest because a moving object is always more easily noticed. If you ride a lot it is a good idea to have your brakes replaced regularly—and use the highest-quality heavy-duty brakes.

If you really like biking, you might also try hanging around a good bike shop for a while to learn how to recognize when things begin to go wrong. A slightly wobbly wheel or loose steering will make your bike perform poorly in an emergency situation. Learning how to prevent these malfunctions before they happen would be valuable.

The proper frame size for your body and proper adjustment of the seat height will improve your riding efficiency and prevent unnecessary tension and pain from riding. For instance, if your frame is too long, it will cause you to lean forward and put your weight on your arms, as well as pressure on your back. Or if your seat is too high, you will strain the outer calf and knee. If it is too low, you can strain your lower back and will not be using the full power of your legs. Also, if your seat is a poor fit you find yourself getting saddle-sore. Get another one, or pad the one you have. Women should make sure they get wider seats that are made for them, because their anatomy is different. For women, properly designed seats are wider in the back and narrower in front.

The way to check the frame size of a man's bike is to straddle the upright bike standing right in front of the seat. To measure the size of a woman's bike, string a piece of masking tape where the bar would be on a man's bike. In both cases you should be able to lift the front of the bike so that the wheel comes off the ground one inch when the bar touches your crotch. To adjust the seat height, sit in the seat with both heels on the pedals. You should be able to backpedal keeping your feet in contact with the pedals. As you come around to the bottom, your knee should straighten. This ensures that when the ball of your foot is on the pedal, your knees will be slightly bent. The center of the ball of your foot should be over the center of the pedal when you are riding. If you are a serious biker, toe clips are a very good idea; they keep your feet properly positioned and, according to cycling studies, allow you to pedal much more efficiently. Toe clips also aid in transmitting force—without toe clips you can pedal for only 70 degrees of the 360-degree arc, but with them you can transmit force to your wheels for a span of 270 degrees. Toe clips also prevent your foot from slipping, especially if you also wear the shoes that lock into the pedals. Toe clips are not for the beginner, who may be fearful of getting stuck in them and falling over.

Efficient bicycling involves maintaining a constant pedaling motion. The function of gears is to make you ride with tremendous efficiency, using the least force to cover the greatest distance. Many people strain their legs and hurt their knees by pedaling in the wrong gear.

If you ride around town, use a bike that allows you to sit erect, one with handlebars tilted up. It is slightly less efficient for riding speed, but it is a lot easier on your lower back, because your bones are in alignment. For distance, and if you don't have a lower-back problem, downward handlebars are usually recommended. To avoid numbing and pain in the heel of the hand, which accompany use of down handlebars, put some padding on your bars. If you still have trouble, the frame is probably too long.

## BOWLING

Bowling is a fairly safe sport, especially if you do it only occasionally. If you're a bowling enthusiast and play often, there are a few things to watch out for.

A common problem is thumb irritation or strain. Friction can occur when the ball is too heavy for you, when your fingers tend to perspire and stick, or when the thumbhole doesn't fit you properly. Get a ball of the proper weight and size for you. Go to a pro shop to get the right ball. They will have a burring drill that custom-fits the hole to your thumb. If you're handy, you can do it yourself with a round file and some sandpaper. If the ball is the right weight and size but your thumb still gets irritated from the friction, get some New-Skin at your local drugstore and paint it on your thumb before you play. That's what the pros do.

Other problems common to bowling are knee pain, lower-back pain, and tennis elbow. Knee problems usually come from poor knee–foot alignment. Check your fitness profile and the alignment chapter to determine if this is the cause of your problem. Knee strain can also result from a poor approach. If the humidity level is high, your feet may tend to stick on your approach, causing knee strain and sometimes a loss of balance. Always check out the approach line. Silicone spray or approach finish, which a good proprietor will have on the premises, will quickly make the floor slick and dry.

Twisting too much when you throw the ball can lead to lower-back and elbow problems. It creates an unnatural strain, almost like throwing a curve in baseball.

A ball that's too heavy for you will also cause you to strain. A good rule of thumb is that the weight of the ball should not throw you out of balance. Always sacrifice weight for balance. If you have good control and direction, you will roll a better game. With a heavy ball you will usually end up in the gutter.

Always do the upper-lower combination warm-up in addition to your general warm-up. If it's easier to do the floor work at home before you go, that's fine. Just finish the warm-up when you get there.

## CANOEING

See **ROWING**

## CLIMBING

See **HIKING**

## DANCE

Every dancer should arrive early and do a preclass warm-up, especially when the class starts in a standing position. In many dance classes, the beginning exercises are not gradual enough or they involve severe stretching. Take extra time to work on those areas of the body which need the most attention. No matter what kind of class you are taking, it is always best to warm up the joints of the legs and feet before they have to support your weight. Fifteen or twenty minutes of warm-up is adequate before a class. Use the general body warm-up Exercises 1 through 17 as your base, and build in your special exercises on top of that. You may want to do some alignment exercises or gentle stretching at the end of your warm-up. Stretch after your class or in the middle of it. Being warmed up is essential.

The class warm-up should begin slowly and gently, increasing the duration and effort of a given exercise gradually. The optimum way of warming up is to start a class lying on the floor, so that there is no pressure on the joints. Repeating the same movements or combinations too many times in a given class fatigues rather than builds muscles and is a most frequent cause of injury in a dance class or rehearsal.

**Tips for Dancer's Tension:** A dancer's most common problem is tension. Here are some tips on how to spot dancer's tension and relieve it:

1. Staring into space while dancing usually indicates head and neck tension and is often accompanied by shallow respiration. In this state, dancers lose contact with the world around them. Sometimes this lack of focus in the eyes is the result of intense internal concentration, but it can also indicate a general spaced-out state. Being out of contact with your body and your surroundings can leave you very vulnerable to injury. In any case, it's no fun watching a dancer with a vacant face. When taking class, try to focus and see other people or objects in the room.

2. When the head is projected forward it shows tension in the neck, shoulders, and upper back. Try the Shoulder Drop exercise, page 72, and the Head Push, page 119. Also, work on improving head-and-neck alignment.

3. Protruding neck muscles are a sign of tension in the jaw, neck, shoulders, upper back, and chest.

4. Gripping the ballet barre with the thumb means tension in the arm and shoulder. The thumb should never touch the barre; it should hang beneath it.

5. Holding up the elbow of the arm that holds the barre produces

tension in the arm and shoulder. Let the elbow of the barre arm drop. The barre should be used for balance and not to hold you up.

6. Constantly contracted buttock muscles show tension in the lower back, abdomen, and pelvic floor and all the muscles of the pelvis and thigh. This is a common error. Your buttock muscles need not be contracted constantly while you are dancing. As a matter of fact, if they are contracted, you severely inhibit the range of movement in your hips and legs.

7. A thigh or calf muscle that is always hard and bulging when not in use signals incorrect use of the legs in movement as well as chronic leg and hip tension. Correctly developed thigh and calf muscles should look long and softly rounded, without any angular definition. One of the best ways to begin reversing this process is daily swimming. Contrary to certain myths, gentle swimming is one of the best exercises for dancers.

8. Raising the heels slightly before beginning a jump or not bringing the heels down to the floor when landing from a jump indicates tension in the feet and legs as well as poor body alignment and an exaggerated turnout. Don't jump more than an inch off the floor before this problem is corrected. It can lead to serious injury. You will generally need help to correct this difficulty. (See Appendix.)

9. Constantly working with too much turnout in the feet is probably the most frequent cause of misalignment, tension, and subsequent injury. It creates tension in the arch, outer foot, shin, calf, thigh, hip, and lower back, and it puts pressure on the ankles, knees, hips, and iliosacral joints. Work with a turnout that you can easily maintain and it will improve gradually. If you turn out far beyond your capacity, you can never build a safe and true turnout.

### Other Tips for Dancers:

1. Try not to dance on a concrete floor or on a wooden one built right over a cement subflooring. Both are unyielding and lead to foot and leg injuries, especially shin splints. If you must, do everything but jump, or jump very low.

2. Don't put a child in pointe shoes too soon. Children's bones are not yet fully formed, and this often leads to irreversible problems. No child should go on toe without at least three years of training, and generally not before twelve years of age.

3. Alignment is the most important aspect of a dancer's safety.

Study the alignment chapter, especially the sections on the knee–foot and pelvic alignment. Find a teacher who has extensive alignment training and work with him or her. This time will be well spent.

4. Always stretch after you are thoroughly warmed up.

5. Don't try to stretch a pulled hamstring. Don't jump with knee pain, shin splints, or ankle or Achilles tendon pain. Your main guide should be, *If it hurts, don't do it*. Stop and wait until you've recovered fully.

6. Dancers should "religiously" take nightly warm baths and elevate their legs.

7. Don't take more than one of the same type of technique class on any given day. It's counterproductive. Never take more than two different dance classes a day.

**A Note for the Dance Teacher:** Teachers are often preoccupied with the care of their students and may neglect themselves, with painful results.

1. Make sure you warm yourself up thoroughly before a class if you demonstrate movements fully when you teach.

2. If you simply indicate or mark movement for the class, don't let yourself get suddenly carried away and do something full out. This is an invitation to injury.

3. Take the advice you give to your students about general body care. Remember that you need to take care of yourself more, rather than less, as you mature.

## FOOTBALL

Football has the highest rate of injury of any sport. Injuries to the ankles and knees occur most often. When your cleats are planted in the ground and you are tackled from the side, your joints are put under a pressure they are unable to absorb. The most common problem is ripped cartilage in the knee. Neck injuries and concussions often occur from head-on impacts or falls. Wrist sprains are also quite common.

Fatigue is also a large factor in football injuries. Training when you're a little tired is all right, but if you're in a game and you feel fatigued, it's best to stop or sit out for a while. Conditioning is the best way to avoid injury. The stronger you are, the less likely it is that you will become fatigued, which is when most injuries occur. Always drink a little water before and during the game. This prevents dehydration and aids in delaying fatigue.

Practicing your own position is the best way to build the strength and know-how that you need. A lineman's needs are different from a quarterback's. Always buy the best equipment you can get and use it. Don't play without it. Be sure to warm up as fully as possible, doing the general and lower-body warm-ups before playing. Jogging and sprinting are a must for football players. If you are flexible as well as strong, you will also be less prone to injury, so stretch regularly.

It's difficult to avoid some injuries in contact sports, but there are some things you can do to minimize the dangers. The most important thing to do when you're tackled is relax and yield. A body that's rigid or brittle gets hurt the most.

## GOLF

Golf is one of the safest sports. The one vulnerable place is the lower back, especially if you like to hit hard with your woods and don't warm up to it.

If you are just starting to golf, begin with the short game; you don't need as much backswing. In golf, it's how you hit the ball, not how hard you hit it. Learn a smooth, easy swing with a follow-through; never pull it short. First learn how to move your hands, shoulders, and hips through. When you force your swing, you stress your lower back—and it usually makes a slice or a hook, which doesn't help your game. Always do the general and upper-body warm-ups before playing. Then work on your swing and your rhythm for ten or fifteen minutes, using your higher irons (7, 8, and 9) first. Then move to your lower irons and finally to your woods before you start your game. If you walk and don't ride the golf cart, it helps to keep your muscles warm.

## GYMNASTICS

The gymnast has many of the same problems as the dancer, with additional hazards of working on the various apparatus. Pulled hamstrings and back pain are quite common, as are broken fingers on the parallel bars. The latter can be avoided if you keep your fingers together when working on the parallel bars. It's a good idea to chalk your hands if they tend to sweat and stick to the bars. Wristbands can also be helpful, in tumbling and vaulting exercises, in protecting you from the impact of landing on your hands.

Unfortunately, gymnastic warm-ups often involve severe stretching instead of proper warm-up followed by stretching. This probably accounts for many of the ankle sprains and knee pains in aerial work — front, back, and twisting flips. Good dance instruction with an accent on alignment in jumping work should be a part of every gymnastic training program.

## HANDBALL

Handball is a fast game with a lot of running, starts, and stops. You need to be extremely warmed up in your upper and lower body before you begin to play. If you volley easily for a long time you will eventually get warm, but a precise warm-up is best. The most common injury is strain at the inner elbow, sometimes referred to medically as golfer's elbow. It is actually a tendinitis at the inner elbow bone. It is most often caused by "hopping" or undercutting the ball, especially before being sufficiently warmed up, and usually happens to hard hitters. Like a baseball pitcher throwing a curveball, if you do it before you are warmed up it puts a great deal of stress on your muscles and you may actually tear the muscle fibers. Other common handball injuries are strain and spasm of the lower back, strained Achilles tendons, and shoulder pain due to either tendon strains or acute bursitis. There are also an occasional sprained ankle and some severe eye injuries, as in racketball.

To protect your hand, always wear a glove. Don't even fool around without one, or you may severely bruise the joints and bones in your hand. Stroking the ball, as the "pros" call it, is the most difficult thing for the beginner to learn. At top speed it looks as if you are hitting the ball, but if you examined this action in slow motion, you would see a relaxed cupped hand catch the ball for an instant and then throw it. You grab it, cradle it, and throw it out toward the wall again in one flowing motion. It should never hurt your hand to hit a handball.

A new device being used more frequently these days to prevent lower-back pain in handball, racketball, and other sports as well is an abbreviated wet suit. Players have skin-diving-equipment shops make a wet suit that runs from the lower rib cage down to the hips. It is about

12 to 14 inches high and about ¼ inch thick. You can have one made for about $10. If you decide to use one of these suits, never wear it for more than twenty to thirty minutes, because it can cause dehydration. Discard it when you begin to feel hot. Also, it should not be too tight. These suits have been helpful to many players with a tendency to lower-back pain.

Eye injuries don't occur in great numbers, but when they do occur they are the most serious. Players are usually hospitalized and often lose some or all of the sight in one eye. In the larger clubs there is usually a serious eye injury at least once a week. Only 5 to 8 percent of the people who play handball wear eye guards, but it is a very good idea to get one for yourself.

## HIKING, MOUNTAIN CLIMBING, AND ROCK CLIMBING

Before hiking or mountain or rock climbing, it's a good idea to warm up. This is especially true if you're carrying a heavy pack. Build your strength gradually by walking around town for an hour or two a day with a weighted backpack for several weeks before your trip. If you jump in too quickly, you will end up injuring your knees, your ankles, and your back, because you weren't ready to absorb the increased load.

## ICE SKATING

Ice skating is a relatively safe activity, especially if you know what you are doing and don't push yourself. The most common injuries are pulled hamstrings and leg cramps. For the beginner, ankle injuries such as sprains or breaks sometimes result from falls. The thing to do when you fall is relax and go with it—never try to catch yourself with your hands, because this can lead to a sprained wrist. The only time to use your hands is to protect your head if you fall forward, but front falls are not as common as backward and side falls, so it is important to learn in these cases how to fall without putting the full impact of your weight onto your arms, hands, and wrists.

The first thing to do to avoid injuries is buy good ice skates. Get the closest fit possible, but don't let the boot crush your toes together. Heavy socks act only as a filler and shouldn't be necessary if the boot is properly fitted. If the boot is too big it is more difficult to balance, and you will tend to wobble and open yourself to tired ankles and injury. Most training is geared toward figure skating, so it is best to buy figure skates. Learn in hockey skates only if your reason for learning is to play hockey. Don't try to learn in racing skates, because they don't give you any support in the ankles.

It is important to put your skates on properly as well. Place your foot in the boot with your heel as far back as possible. Align your knee and ankle so that they are vertical and your foot is straight forward. If you lace your boot in the wrong position, that's the stance you will be in when you stand up, making it more difficult to start skating. Lace your boot tightly and snugly across the arch, but not across the ankle. If it is too tight at the top, it will cut off your blood circulation.

Always warm up before you put on your skates. Warm-up on the ice is difficult, to say the least! Stretching is not essential to the warm-up, but may be included if you like. It is more important to stretch after you finish skating, especially the back of your legs.

## KARATE

It is difficult to make generalized statements about the martial arts as practiced in the United States because there is such a wide range of teaching and training styles and methods. The caliber of the training has a great deal to do with the later possibility of injury, and the quality of the instructor, his attitudes and skills, will determine this. If you are trained in the traditional style in which you have to be "tough as nails" and constantly prove your manhood, the likelihood of injury is tremendously high. If, on the other hand, you approach the sport slowly and with caution, you can be relatively safe from injury.

American karate differs from the traditional style of karate in that the American school insists on no actual physical contact in the first three to six months of training. Dummies and kicking bags are used. There is no "breaking of boards" to toughen up the hand by creating tremendous amounts of scar tissue. Hand conditioning of this nature is unnecessary in modern-day self-defense. When these martial arts originated, one had to be able to punch through metal armor in battle. Since this is no longer necessary, I suggest that you stay away from hitting trees and rocks! Hitting anything with your hand can cause wrist injuries if the bones of the wrist and arm are not lined up properly. This can be avoided with some training and practice.

Of the many leg injuries in karate, pain in the knee and pulled hamstrings and groin muscles are the most common. There are also a fair number of lower-back injuries, especially with beginners. The most important thing is to learn how to fall and roll properly to protect your back. One of the main causes of knee problems is incorrect kicking form. Do not kick flat-footed. Rise up onto the ball of your foot and pivot every time you kick, especially if you have a tendency toward knee problems. Pulled-muscle injuries are often the result of kicking before you've had an adequate warm-up. The warm-up included in most karate training is stretching. As we've seen in Chapter 7, this approach can be dangerous. It will eventually warm you up, but at the expense of weakening your ligaments and tendons. It is better to do a thorough upper- and lower-body warm-up before you begin your class.

The most important thing is to have a good instructor. If you see beginners sparring freely or doing push-ups on their knuckles or if there is a general tone of bravado and the teaching has a "pushy" quality to it—find another school.

## KAYAKING

See **ROWING**

## PLATFORM TENNIS

This popular new game sweeping the East and moving West has all the hazards and cautions of tennis, so refer to that section of this chapter. The heavier racket increases the risk of injury when there is unnecessary tension or poor form. If you have a tendency to get tennis elbow, try switching to racketball, which offers less chance of injury.

## RACKETBALL

Racketball is deceptive; it takes more energy than you think it does. You need strength and flexibility in order to be able to lunge into all kinds of positions. It's important to be quite warmed up before you begin, because of the sudden quick starts and stops that are a part of the game. Most people who play racketball usually don't warm up. This is probably a major cause of injuries in this particular sport.

The most common injuries in racketball are tennis elbow and generalized arm and shoulder pain. These injuries are often caused by poor backhand form, such as meeting the ball behind the center of your body instead of in line with your lead foot. Other common injuries are lower-back pain, pulled hamstrings, and strained Achilles tendons. Be sure to warm up your upper and lower body thoroughly before you play.

There are a great many people who suffer severe retina damage from getting hit in the eye with the ball. The pros feel that eye guards should be mandatory for racketball.

## ROLLER SKATING

Roller skating is one of the safest sports activities. As with ice skating, most of the injuries that occur are from not knowing how to fall, and the worst that happens is a skinned elbow or knee, or a few bruises.

Everyone falls sometimes — even a professional — and more serious injuries can occur. It is possible to break an ankle or leg, and some skaters injure their tailbone by stiffening when they fall backward. When you fall, just draw your arms across your chest or belly, bend your knees, bring your feet together, and allow yourself to slide or roll. Try to relax. This, of course, is easier said than done, and you might try practicing falls on a rug or some mats.

Good skates of the proper fit and adjustment are vital to safe skating. The boot should be firmly fitted so that it won't rub and give you blisters. The lacing, similar to that in ice skating, should be tight over the instep and a little looser at the ankle. The wheel-assembly, or truck, adjustment must be precise in order to give you the right amount of flexibility, so that you can turn and maneuver easily. The more control you have, the safer you will be.

The safest place to skate is in a roller rink. If you skate outdoors, which is certainly a lovely thing to do, the risks of accident and injury increase. Gravel, cracks, dirt, wetness, and people are no longer under your control, so you must be very alert and aware when you skate outdoors.

A light general and lower-body warm-up is advisable before roller skating.

## ROWING, CANOEING, KAYAKING

Rowing can be a very strenuous activity if you row competitively or in white water. Build up your strength slowly to avoid strains and sore muscles, and do the general and upper-body warm-ups for these sports.

Canoeing on a lake is relatively safe, but it is wise to wear a life jacket, especially if you're not a terrific swimmer. Canoeing in white water (rapids) can be dangerous if you are not skilled at both canoeing and reading the river. The following safety advice for kayaking also applies to canoeing.

Kayaking can be very dangerous, so it is important to be schooled properly in river safety, in learning how to read the water, and in maneuvering. There are hard-shell and inflatable kayaks. The hard-shell variety gives you greater maneuverability and control, once you have the basic skill mastered. A one-week course is usually enough time to learn the basics, but real skill is acquired only after several years of practice. When hard-shell kayaking, always wear a life jacket, a helmet, and the proper clothing for the temperature of the water— e.g., a wet suit.

Operating an inflatable kayak is easier and less hazardous than operating a hard-shell kayak. A helmet is not necessary, but a life jacket is. A short boat is less maneuverable than a long one—one person can maneuver a 11½-foot boat much more easily than a 9½-foot boat. You ride higher in the water and can move in a straight line with greater ease. Normally you sit in the middle of the boat, but if your boat twists from side to side or if you are in a headwind, greater safety and maneuverability is gained from moving forward. For a tail wind, you should move slightly toward the rear of the kayak.

For the greatest control, buy paddles with straight blades. Curved paddles hinder back-paddling strokes. Always feather the paddles at 90 degrees to each other. This minimizes and almost eliminates wind resistance against the paddle that is out of the water. There are four or five essential strokes that must be mastered—one for cruising, one that will increase your speed, another that will allow you to move sideways quickly to miss a rock, and others that will slow you down. Always scout a rapid that you are not familiar with, and accumulate as much information as you can about the river before you take a run. There are excellent white-water guides for almost every river.

Never tie your bags or equipment to your inflatable kayak, as this might make it difficult to turn your boat back over if you fall out and your boat turns over, or dumps, as it is called. Always place your supplies in waterproof plastic bags, which you can purchase at any good supply store. If you do dump, hold on to your paddle, but let go of your boat. The only time to hold on to the boat is if you are in a boil (an underwater current that pulls you down). Tuck your knees up toward your chest and keep your feet out in front of you, so that you will be able to bounce off and negotiate the rocks as you come to them. If you go down the river backward or if you let your feet dangle below, they may get caught between two rocks and you would be trapped. You should wear sneakers or similar footwear to protect your feet. It is also important to steer clear of fallen dead trees; they are dangerous.

Always kayak in a group of at least three people, one or more of whom have experience. If you get pinned under a rock, one person may not be strong enough to pull you out. If you wear eyeglasses, get shatterproof safety glasses or ones made out of plastic. Always have them secured with a special elastic guard, easily purchased at a drugstore.

The most dangerous time to kayak is in the spring, when the rivers are high or flooded and extremely cold. This is when most fatal accidents occur. The most common injuries in kayaking are tendinitis, which can occur at the back of the wrist or the elbow, and dislocation of the shoulder. Wrist and elbow problems generally result from failure to keep the wrist straight and also from too much tension. The beginning student usually squeezes the paddle too hard and over-tenses his muscles, and often does too much too soon. When technique is good, the fingers are relaxed and there is a balance of push with the upper hand and pull with the lower hand. The motion is relaxed and strong—not straining.

## RUNNING

*Always do warm-up exercises before you run.* The different exercises you do should remain constant throughout the year, but the length of time you spend on them should be adjusted to correspond with the season, the temperature, and the vulnerable areas of your body. For instance, if you run outdoors when it's cold, warm up for a longer period of time. If you have knee problems, spend more time on the floor warming up your joints before standing up. In the event that you can't warm up fully, jog very slowly with your feet barely leaving the ground for the first five to ten minutes before picking up any speed. Do your daily running, as opposed to racing, at a comfortable speed. You should be able to talk and have a conversation while you run. If you can't, you are running too fast. Slow down.

Running shoes are very important. Be sure they fit properly and have thick-layered, cushioned heels and soles. Heavy runners who come down hard on their feet should buy the thickest-heeled shoes available. They should also put 2-inch Dr. Scholl Inner Soles in each shoe.

Make sure your shoes are wide enough to be comfortable for your toes. If the front is too narrow or pointed for your foot, it increases the likelihood of injury, because the ball of the foot cannot naturally expand when you step on it. This can cause the foot to cramp. When your shoes get worn out a bit, wear an extra pair of socks to ensure a firm fit, but replace them as soon as you can. It isn't good to run in shoes that are very stretched out or worn down unevenly on the bottom, because this creates an unbalanced running form. So if you run a good deal, buy shoes fairly often. Also, it's a good idea to tape your laces onto your shoes with a small piece of adhesive tape if you do any distance running or sprinting. *Don't run in sneakers.* They don't offer adequate support or enough cushion for distance running. Also, make it a habit to wear white socks. The dye in colored socks comes off on the feet and infects cuts and blisters.

The safest running surfaces for your legs are earth and grass; the next-safest are padded indoor tracks. These absorb some of the shock to the legs. Concrete is the worst surface to run on, because running on concrete aggravates any vulnerabilities to injury. If you run on concrete, run slowly and low to the ground to minimize the impact. Tar and asphalt surfaces are better than concrete.

Running barefoot on beach sand is dangerous. Never run barefoot on soft sand, except for some spontaneous fooling around. The movement of the sand interferes with your traction and balance, making it easy to sprain a muscle in your foot or injure your Achilles tendon or ankle. If you want to run barefoot on the beach, do it next to or even slightly in the water. A flat part of the wet sand is better for running than an incline. Don't run with one side on a downhill slant.

Don't jog downhill. Walk, or run full speed. If the incline is very slight, jogging is okay. Be careful in the fall if you run on ground covered with leaves—a lot of ankles are sprained on hidden holes and rocks.

The body must adjust itself to an unaccustomed running surface. A sudden change in your regular running surface, even if it's from asphalt to earth, warrants cutting your running time in half for three or four days to allow your body to readjust to avoid injury.

If your calves and legs tested out as very tense in your fitness profile, you should probably spend as much time as necessary learning how to relax them; otherwise you'll be quite prone to running injuries. Also, runners who have poor alignment of the ankle, knee, or pelvis constantly risk injury. Running with the feet turned out stresses the ankle and knee, and with a swayback, every step adds stress to the lower back. Orthotics can be helpful for these problems.

Recently devised scientific tests have determined that a person weighing 120 pounds absorbs about 1,000 pounds of pressure throughout his body with each step. Ideally, this impact should go through your whole body. It becomes a problem when a part of the body is out of line and the tension is absorbed by the weakest link. The impact is also affected by how heavily you run. If you rattle the china every time you walk across the kitchen, you're probably a heavy runner. Try to run with the feeling that you're floating and barely touching the ground. Roll through your feet from heel to toe. Don't slam down on your heel; land softly. Don't run flat-footed, and as you are running, try to keep your feet and knees parallel. Your alignment test should tell you if you're capable of this.

If you get tight in your shoulders or arms, do some exercises while you run. First raise and lower your shoulders as in the Shoulder Drop exercise (page 72). Shake your hands vigorously, moving them out to the side and even above your head. Clasp one hand after the other into a tight fist and then release it. Try not to grip your elbows into the sides of your body; imagine there is a softly inflated, round rubber balloon in each of your armpits.

## SAILING

Crewing a sailboat can be hard work, often resulting in shoulder, neck, and lower-back pain and sometimes in shin splints. You often have to sit in one position with your head twisted awkwardly for quite a while. A good way to keep from tightening up is to keep your body moving where you can.

If you're racing, try to find a comfortable hiking position. If you're in a bad position and you are straining your legs, you may get shin splints. You will invariably build up tension if you're keeling a lot and bracing with your foot to keep from falling. Shake your legs out intermittently and stamp a few times whenever you can to discharge some of the tension.

If you are steering, fighting the wind with your tiller arm can also build tension. Switch arms as often as you can, and do the shoulder and arm tension-releasing exercises. You can accumulate tension in your face and head from glare. Always wear a hat with a brim or sunglasses, if the glare is very intense.

Sailing is primarily an upper-body activity. You should do the full general warm-up and the upper-body warm-up, accenting the shoulder exercises. It's a good idea to balance out your body by doing some swimming or running after you finish sailing.

## SKIING, CROSS-COUNTRY

Cross-country skiing is different from downhill skiing and requires more exertion and a pulling action in your upper body. It is a relatively safe sport, although leg strains and knee pains occur sometimes. Do the full warm-ups for the upper body as well as the lower body.

The most important things to know for your safety are, first, to be familiar with the weather conditions and, second, to have a realistic perspective on your strengths and abilities. Getting caught in a bad storm or pushing your limits and being 4 miles from nowhere and extremely tired can be dangerous. The most hazardous time on cross-country skis is when there is a whiteout. This occurs through a combination of fog, wind, and snow. I have had skiers tell me that when this happens, they could not see their own feet!

The clothes you wear for cross-country skiing are different from those you would wear for downhill skiing, because you work much harder and build up a tremendous body heat. Layer your clothing as in downhill skiing, but don't wear windproof and waterproof clothing like a parka or warm-up pants, because you will get too hot. Wool is usually a good choice. Wear a small day pack so that you can remove or replace clothing as your body temperature changes. For instance, you can become extremely hot, or you may get stranded and need to stay warm for an extended period of time. Always ski with at least one other person in case one of you gets hurt and the other needs to go for help.

## SKIING, DOWNHILL

Since skiing is a seasonal sport for most people, ski safely by preparing your legs for four to six weeks before the season begins. Do the general body and lower-body warm-ups followed by the leg-strengthening exercises, three or four times per week. If you are somewhat inflexible, do the stretch series after the strength-building exercises. If you find strengthening exercises boring, then jog, increasing slowly to about 2 miles over a six-week period.

The knee is the part of the body most frequently injured in skiing. Two common contributing factors are tension and poor alignment—having tense legs or turned-in knees greatly increases your chance of injury. It makes a difference if you can get these problems straightened out, so try the exercises for tense legs (page 129) or misaligned knees (page 193–98).

Always warm up before you ski. Do the general body warm-up in your room before you go to the slopes; then finish in the lodge before you put on your ski boots. It is especially important to warm up effectively when it's very cold. Don't be concerned about appearing foolish doing your lower-body warm-up. Soon everybody will be doing it! Accent the parts of your body that need the most warming up. The entire warm-up should take between ten and twelve minutes.

Staying warmed up depends on how busy the slope is. If there's a half-hour wait at the chair lift, you'll have to work to keep your muscles and joints warm. The wait in line and the chairlift ride are times when your muscles begin to contract and stiffen.

While in line, lift your legs and walk in place for a few seconds every minute or so. Then tighten and relax your thigh muscles. Hold each contraction for about a second. Now alternately tighten and relax your buttock muscles. Do some Shoulder Rolls, Shoulder Drops, and Side Reaches (see pages 71–72). Contract and relax your toes (that's if you can still feel them).

While on the chair lift, alternate raising and lowering each leg a few inches off the seat. Also, gently swing your legs forward and back, bending at the knee. Keep moving your shoulders periodically. Make a pulsing fist with both hands, gripping and releasing your poles.

Good boots and bindings are your most important asset. Don't buy cheap or uncomfortable equipment. You can find an excellent guide to high-quality boots in Skiing Magazine.* I also recommended that

* Michael W. Chapman, M.D., "Ski Boots, How To Make Sure They Fit," Skiing Magazine (October 1975): 96.

you buy the best bindings you can, and always make sure that they are working properly. If you are a beginner, take the time to learn how to adjust and test your bindings. Bend your knees forward abruptly to see if they release. They should also release when you move forcefully from side to side. Get a pair of Ski Stops, new safety devices that prevent runaway skis when you fall. When your skis come off, the Ski Stops make them stick in the snow where you lost them. They eliminate the strap that keeps the ski attached to your leg during the fall. When the ski is strapped to you, it often gets tangled up and can hit you — in the head.

Most skiing injuries are sustained by beginners and budding intermediates who attempt challenges they're not ready for. Skill is vitally important in skiing. Knowing how to stop and how to fall can save you from a torn cartilage or broken leg. Skiers who take lessons and become truly skillful suffer fewer injuries. Speed is a constant danger. Resist it. Without skill it can lead to disaster. Don't go faster than what you can handle.

Never ski when you're tired. It is quite dangerous when your reaction time slows down by even one second. Always quit when you're tired.

Beginners should not try night skiing. It is more dangerous unless you are quite skillful.

If you're going to ski for a week, don't start out like "gangbusters." Do the least amount of skiing that first day. Add about a half-hour onto each of the following days. Preparing in the off-season will allow you to ski longer, faster. And remember: You *can't* begin this season at the same level at which you ended the last one.

One of the greatest dangers in skiing is finding yourself on top of a slope that is too advanced for you to ski safely. The grading of the slopes may vary from place to place. Find out what slopes are best for you by asking someone who should know. A fellow skier is often not the best source for this information. What's an easy intermediate slope to her might not be so easy for you (or might even be a terrifying experience for you).

When you are falling, relax. Don't stiffen your body. Remember to drop your poles, because the easiest way to break your wrist is to hold on to them. When getting up from a fall, make sure your skis are under you and pointing up the mountain. It's a simple rule, but many often forget it. If the slopes are extremely icy and dangerous, I suggest reading instead of skiing. Find a friend, a cozy fire, or a sauna.

It's best to wear several layers of thin, high-quality ski apparel which maximize your freedom of movement. What keeps you warm is the heat trapped between the layers of clothing. For example, two pairs of regular socks are better than one pair of thick ones. You'll barely feel the cold while skiing if you are dressed properly and the weather is not unreasonably cold. Buy the best, because it's well worth the expense. When your body is wet and it's freezing out, your cold muscles will contract. This makes you quite vulnerable to being injured. All the warm-ups in the world won't help you in this situation.

A thorough warm-up; good equipment; warm, light clothing; good form and skill; and a little common sense all lessen the risks of being injured. Together they provide the best possible protection.

## SOCCER

Soccer is a demanding sport. It involves the constant motions of sprinting, twisting, and turning. As in football, most injuries occur through fatigue and exhaustion, so the more endurance you develop, the better your chance of remaining free of injury will be. Professionals are often hurt because they suffer from tension coupled with fatigue. In addition, when they are injured, they rarely sit out long enough to heal.

Soccer's most common injuries are ankle sprains, broken feet and ankles, leg cramps, shin splints, and contact injuries from being kicked or stepped on. Do the general body warm-up and lower-body warm-up, followed by jogging, before you play. Make sure you have the proper equipment—never use tennis or street shoes for soccer. Wear the inexpensive molded-plastic-cleat shoes. If you are a serious player, also wear shin guards.

## SOFTBALL

See **BASEBALL AND SOFTBALL**

## SQUASH

Squash can be a fast or a slow game, depending on how competitively you play it. After people get into it, they usually play very vigorously. It is usually said that one hour of squash is like two hours of tennis. The most frequent accident in squash is being hit with the racket, usually on the head or on the elbow. If you wear glasses, it's a good idea to get the rubber-and-steel eyeglass protectors. If you play a fast game of squash, the most likely place you'll be injured is your ankle or knee and possibly your lower back. You may have to twist and turn with great speed. If you are a beginner at squash, play only fifteen to thirty minutes at first. A thorough warm-up, both upper- and lower-body, is a must before squash.

## TENNIS

Always warm up before you play tennis. It will reduce the risk of injury, and it will also improve your game. If you don't warm up, your body will fatigue more quickly and over the years you will become more vulnerable to injury.

Tennis is a sport that involves both the upper and the lower body. Do the general body warm-up first, then the upper-/lower-body combination warm-up. But learn the complete upper- and lower-body warm-ups anyway, in case you need them. Feel free to change the warm-up combination to suit your needs. If you play very easily for at least the first ten minutes, you may not need to do as much of the lower-body warm-up. Spend more time preparing your upper body if you've had tennis elbow or a shoulder injury in the past.

Tennis is a very demanding sport, and here are some very basic hints for safety while playing. *Once you've hit the ball, always loosen your grasp on the racket.* Consistently squeezing the grip of the handle produces fatigue and excess muscle tension. Be especially careful not to squeeze with your small and ring fingers. This frequently contributes to tennis elbow.

*Make sure you get a racket of the right weight, balance and size for your hand.* An undersized grip makes the smaller fingers unstable, a common problem among women players. If you must choose between an undersized and an oversized racket for a particular game, take the one that's a little too big. Some players have a tendency to whip light rackets, which strains their wrists. If your hands sweat a lot and slip, you may have to hold the racket too tightly, expending much more energy than necessary. This may lead to tension buildup and fatigue, and you can solve it by putting rosin or a layer of tennis gauze on the grip. You can also build up the bottom of the grip with gauze to prevent your hand from slipping down.

*How you hold the racket is crucial.* Your hold should allow the force of impact to pass through your whole arm and into your body. When the racket slips or when you play with bad form—for instance, using a lot of wrist movement—the full impact often falls on a joint or tendon, repeatedly stressing it, which results in injury.

People with bad knees must take certain precautions. Clay courts are best, because they reduce the shock absorbed by the legs. *Always wear good tennis shoes with enough padding to absorb the ground shock*, especially on hard courts.

If you are recovering from a back problem, be careful when you serve. Arching way back can trigger another injury. You pick up the ball hundreds of times in an hour in tennis—do it correctly to avoid lower-back strain and injury. Never bend from the waist with your legs straight. The safest way to retrieve the ball is to place it between your heel and tennis racket and lift it up. Get good at this technique and save a lot of energy. Don't rush to pick up a ball out of play; save your energy for the game.

It makes a difference if you take a break every thirty or forty minutes, resting for three to four minutes. You will last a lot longer on the court. Walk around a bit, and drink some water. If you feel a little tight in the legs, lie down and do some Foot-Shaking (page 53). If your arms and upper body feel stiff, do some Arm Circles (page 87) and Hand-Shaking (page 73). It will stimulate your blood flow and might give you a boost of energy. I know my suggestion is not in keeping with the rules of the game, but I have seen enough strained tendons, joint pain, and back and other injuries to assure me that my idea is a good one.

One of the drawbacks of tennis is that it builds up the muscles on one side of your body. This unbalanced muscular strength pulls unevenly on the spine, often resulting in a number of problems including shoulder pain and lower-back pain. It would be ideal for people to learn from the start to play ambidextrously, but unfortunately this is usually unrealistic and impractical. If you are a beginner, learn to hit holding the racket with two hands, especially on the backhand. This allows you to use both sets of muscles. It's easy to switch to one hand later on, if you like. If this sounds ridiculous, get into the habit of volleying with your other arm.

If you have tennis elbow and love the game, muster as much self-control as possible. The urge to get back into play can be deadly. Recently, I had a client with tennis elbow, who came to me after suffering with it for six months. He complained that it kept flaring up, usually after a day or two of playing. He said, "I rest for four or five days, play, and then it comes right back again, but it's not too bad." He had seen a doctor who had instructed him to rest for a month or two. My client thought this was unreasonable, because his elbow would stop hurting after only three or four days of rest.

At our first meeting, I found that his shoulder and arm were as hard as a rock. I had him swing his racket, to show me how he used his arm. I also learned that his warm-up consisted of Push-ups, Sit-ups, and Running in Place. I told him that I'd work with him only if he'd follow all my instructions.

Working with him twice a week helped him to reduce a lot of tension in his arm and shoulder. I instructed him not to play tennis until further notice. In addition, I asked him to take warm baths every day, and to put ice on the painful area three times a day. After a week of this routine, I got him swimming every other day and taught him the warm-ups. To maintain his cardiovascular fitness and general strength, I had him running three or four times a week.

The third week of our work was rough going. He insisted that he was fine, and he wanted to return to the court immediately. He said, "I'll come three times a week for treatment, if I could start playing again." I explained that he had only just begun to heal, and that returning to play too soon would result in retearing the muscle fibers or the tendon.

My explanation was not convincing enough. He insisted, "But I feel better than the other times I returned to the courts. If I get back to it slow and easy, I'm sure I won't blow all our work." Redoubling my efforts, I explained, "Had I worked with you when you first injured yourself, or even after the first relapse, it might have taken only a few weeks to get you back to playing. But after several reinjuries, plus the tension in your arm, it will take at least another two weeks. Now we have to slowly recondition your arm with planned exercises."

The discussion was on Friday. Monday morning, not entirely surprised, I received a frantic call. "I did it. You warned me, but I did it. Tell me what to do. This time I'll listen." Within six weeks he was back on the court. This time he didn't reinjure himself.

## VOLLEYBALL

Volleyball can be a vigorous sport, so your arms and legs should be thoroughly warmed up before you start to play. Being in top physical condition reduces the likelihood of injury, and building your endurance through running is an excellent way to prepare yourself for this sport. If you play volleyball only part of the year, it's a good idea to start conditioning yourself five to six weeks ahead of time so that your body will be ready to get right into it when the time comes.

Improper contact between the hand and the ball can cause jammed fingers, especially for beginning players. For the more advanced player, ankle sprains, knee injuries, and shin splints are more common, as are strains in the shoulder and upper arm from an overdone or incorrect spike of the ball. Contusions to the hipbone can occur when a player is diving for the ball. If you are thin and want to protect your hipbones, wear hip pads. In addition, if you are playing on a wood floor indoors always wear knee pads to avoid floor burns during a bump or pass. Heel contact and good alignment are essential in jumping during volleyball to avoid shin splints and ankle injuries.

## WARMING UP FOR
## YOUR EVERYDAY ACTIVITIES

People get injured doing all sorts of activities that they don't think of as exercise. Many professions, hobbies, and seemingly ordinary activities require great physical effort. Other activities can become straining and intense if we do them for a long time.

Your body needs warm-up preparation for such activities as playing a musical instrument, raking leaves, moving furniture, digging ditches, heavy carpentry, construction work, gardening, shoveling snow. If your job involves strenuous activity, you might benefit from warming up each morning before you go to work.

You should be especially conscientious about warming up if certain parts of your body are weak or vulnerable due to previous injury. If you tend to feel lower-back pain or knee pain, don't suddenly run for the bus on a cold winter morning or offer to push a car stuck in the snow. This kind of spontaneity can blow your ski vacation and give you pain for a couple of months.

Clients often walk into my office with muscle strains and pain from such seemingly innocent acts as raking their front lawn, shoveling snow, or even playing their violin. They express shock that they are so out of shape that a little strain could create such a problem. I explain to them that though being in shape is sometimes a factor, such injuries are usually caused by their muscles' being cold when they began their activity.

**Gardening:** In the summer I see as many people with back problems from gardening as I do from any sports injury. Before you garden, always warm up. Do it outside. When you plant and especially when you weed, work on your knees or in a sitting position. Never garden constantly bent over from a standing position. That is the surest way of getting injured. The upper-body warm-up is what's important here. Take frequent breaks, and do some of the upper-body warm-ups again.

**House Cleaning:** Many people injure themselves simply cleaning their houses. Housecleaning can be very strenuous, especially if you try to do a thorough job and move furniture to clean behind it. Cleaning is an activity that requires both an upper- and lower-body warm-up, so do the combination warm-up. Be careful never to lean over furniture to lift something or to open a window. Always get right up close. When mopping the floor, try to keep a straight back. If you scrub the floor on your hands and knees, placing a pillow under your knees will protect them.

**Taxi Drivers, Truck Drivers, and Traveling Salesmen:** If you drive a truck or car all day long your spine gets bounced around a lot. You probably sit in a collapsed position, which compresses your spine. A simple way to compensate for this is to always drive with a pillow behind your back or to get a removable orthopedic seat made just for you. This gives added support and helps take pressure off your lower back. Sitting collapsed like this often leads to lower-back pain, disc problems, and numbness in the legs.

If you can, it's best to stop every hour or so, get out, and do a few standing warm-ups or just move around. Even if it's just for a couple of minutes, it will do your body a world of good. Once a day, be sure to do the full warm-ups and an activity that gets you moving your lower body, such as running—it's easy to do anywhere.

**Moving, Movers, and Air-Conditioner Installers:** Moving heavy furniture by yourself is the fastest way to back pain that I know of. If you're going to move, call a mover. Knowing how to move furniture is a skill and should not be thought of lightly, especially if you're over thirty-five or if you've had a previous back or shoulder injury. Movers know their job and know how to lift things with the least effort and the most safety. Always lift with your legs, not with your back. The heavier the object, the more upright your back should be. Movers and air-conditioner installers should warm up each morning before they go to work.

**Sanitation Workers, Construction Workers, House Painters, and Plumbers:** All of these professions are hard on the lower back. Maintaining your strength in this part of the body is as important as adequate warm-up preparation. If you are out of work or on vacation for more than a week, which is common in the construction industry, it's good to try to maintain the strength of your back with vigorous exercise or by playing a sport regularly. Know where your weak spots are and be sure to warm up those areas the most thoroughly each day before going to work.

**Going Out Dancing:** If you are the kind of disco dancer who moves real slowly and takes his time getting into it, you probably don't need a warm-up; you get it by starting slowly. But if you're the kind of person that throws himself into it in a big way, a general warm-up just before you go out dancing is a good idea.

**Digging, Shoveling, and Raking:** These are three activities that are deceptively difficult. Whether shoveling snow or digging ditches or raking the leaves on your lawn, always warm up. Pay special attention to your lower back. When you dig or shovel, lift and throw with a straight back. Dirt and snow can be very heavy.

**Playing an Instrument:** Musicians are a large group of people who frequently get injured. In fact, musicians, particularly the younger ones, suffer from nearly as many pains and injuries as athletes do, amazing as that may seem. They don't think of their profession or their hobby as exercise, but they need both warm-up preparation and exercise breaks to use parts of their bodies that remain very still for many hours.

The major problem musicians have is the unavoidable repetition of the same movements for long periods of time. Sometimes they sit or stand in one position for ten or twelve hours a day. This creates tension and fatigue, which is inevitable even with the best training. Half of a musician's practice time is spent battling fatigue and tension. Two three-hour sessions per day would be quite sufficient, if musicians learned how to move and breathe properly.

Your mind and body can only absorb so much at one time. After a certain point, your brain goes on what we could call "circuit overload," and all you do is fight yourself. Taking breaks and working for reasonable amounts of time will make the musician learn faster, not slower.

Each musical instrument also presents its own problems. One violinist I worked with always favored her right leg. She had suffered back pain on the right side of her body for two years. A second violinist tightened his chin and neck and always held his breath on difficult passages. A cellist I helped a year ago always kept her heels raised slightly off the floor. This small error in body posture caused her to suffer cramps in her calves and lower-back discomfort.

I recommend that musicians and other professionals who sit for prolonged periods get other kinds of exercise regularly—at least three times a week. Running and swimming are generally the best. *The two cardinal rules for musicians should be to warm up before practicing and to take frequent breaks.* Do the general warm-up and the upper-body warm-up, especially Arm Circles (see page 87). If you are practicing at home, take a short bath or shower during one or even two of your breaks. Take a five- to ten-minute break about every forty-five minutes, and never practice more than two-and-a-half to three hours without a prolonged break. A low back cushion is a must.

I often suggest that musicians sing or make sounds while they are practicing. This encourages better breathing. It's also helpful to place a small cork between your teeth. Cut a piece of cork about a half-inch thick from your next wine bottle. Hold the cork between your teeth, keeping most of it outside your mouth. It helps you breathe and relax your jaw. If you bite through the cork while you are playing, then jaw tension is one of your problems. Some musicians are amazed when they bite through their first cork in a few minutes. See if you can spot your tension and see the tension-relaxation chapter for suggestions on what to do about it.

# APPENDIX

There are several very effective therapeutic methods and techniques in current use for working with the body. Some work primarily with postural alignment and movement habits, others primarily with the removal of excess tension, but all have in common the use of imagery for dealing with problems of bodily structure and movement.

The originators of the use of Imagery in working with postural alignment, movement, and exercise were F. M. Alexander, the creator of the Alexander Technique, and Mabel Todd, the author of *The Thinking Body*, (Brooklyn, N.Y.: Dance Horizons, 1937).

## THE ALEXANDER TECHNIQUE

In the early 1900s, F. M. Alexander became the first person to use mental images to correct body movement and posture. An aspiring actor who suffered from the frequent and complete loss of his voice, Alexander was desperate to find help. He sought treatment from medical professionals, but his condition didn't improve. This motivated him to experiment on his own. By studying himself in a mirror, Alexander discovered new approaches to his problem. Eventually, his experimentation led to his complete cure, and to a series of innovative techniques to correct the body's alignment during movement by using the mind's power to inhibit inappropriate muscle action. He developed a collection of images or "non-doing" directives which helped to release and lengthen different parts of the body. He used these to reeducate the body in performing such everyday movements as sitting down, standing, and walking. These techniques are quite powerful and have had a profound effect on the lives of many people.

His training reestablishes correct alignment to a point where it becomes automatic. Others have subsequently borrowed from and adapted many of Alexander's ideas and techniques. His method, known as the Alexander Technique, works to create an economy of movement (moving with minimal tension), better postural alignment and balance in order to free your energy. Students learn to move in a relaxed and easy manner. Generally this reeducation process takes between six months and a year. Training to be an Alexander teacher extends over two-and-a-half years, at which time students are graduated and certified. There are practitioners throughout the United States, England, and Australia. The Alexander Technique is widely known and has been used especially by those in the performing arts.

## MABEL TODD'S BASIC PRINCIPLES
## OF NATURAL POSTURE

Though a contemporary of Alexander's, Mabel Todd independently developed her own revolutionary approaches to movement, postural alignment, and exercise. She and Alexander only became aware of each other's work many years after they were both established.

As a young woman in the early 1900s, Mable Todd severely injured her back from a fall. The best doctors of her day told her she would never walk again. Rejecting this pessimistic diagnosis, Miss Todd struggled for years to regain her health, and did so. She worked on her body spontaneously with visualization techniques to teach herself how to move again. Her personal struggles led her, years later, to create her method, which she called "the Basic Principles of Natural Posture." In developing her theories she studied physics, biology, architecture, engineering, and everything known about posture at that time. While studying for a degree in speech at Emerson College of Oratory in Boston, she saw that some of her fellow students' speech difficulties were due to poor posture. She discovered this was particularly true when the head and neck posture was poor. Years later, she began to work with her contemporaries to try to help them. She soon found that most people moved incorrectly, and developed techniques using Imagery, as she had on herself, to help people change their body posture and movement habits. These anatomically accurate and relaxing images became the backbone of her approach.

As her career progressed, Miss Todd had private practices in New York and Boston, where she worked with people who suffered from pain due to weakness, injury, and muscular imbalance. These rehabilitative efforts comprised her life's work.

Mabel Todd did not develop her therapeutic methods into an established system to be passed on to other practitioners, but two of her students, Dr. Lulu Sweigard and Barbara Clark, continued to develop her work in new directions.

**Lulu Sweigard:** Dr. Lulu Sweigard, author of *Human Movement Potential*,\* was the first person to systematize the therapeutic use of Imagery. She called her approach Ideo-Kinetic Facilitation. She spent years studying neuroanatomy to find out exactly what happens in the nervous system when you use an image to change posture. She did posture-research studies at Columbia and New York universities with people who had different postural problems to see what occurred when the body was brought into proper anatomical balance and alignment through the use of imagined movement. Precise measurements and X-rays were used to document the changes. When her subjects' bodies came closer to anatomical balance, the same changes occurred in all of them. They got a little taller; high, tight shoulders dropped spontaneously and widened across the back; pushed-forward ribs relaxed downward, and so forth. Dr. Sweigard developed and refined hundreds of specific images that are extremely effective.

**Barbara Clark:** Barbara Clark became a student of Mabel Todd's after completing her education in nursing. Clark began her work by

---

\**Human Movement Potential: Ideo-Kinetic Facilitation*, New York: Harper & Row, 1974.

relating Todd's approach to the special needs of children. She developed imagery and stories which helped children to experience postural change, and designed special toys and games which fostered the development of sound movement habits. Later, she worked with dancers and began to draw and write. In her drawings, she tried to create visual imagery in which the direction of postural change was clearly expressed as well as the sense of balance, ease, and rhythm characteristic of the well-aligned body. These image drawings were the focus of lessons which Miss Clark organized into three "body-alignment" manuals. Like Mabel Todd, Barbara Clark never formally named her work or specified a system for teaching it. Her thrust was to simplify Todd's ideas through the development of several image patterns applicable to many of the body's joints and to enlist the creative participation of her students in an effort to make the principles of skeletal alignment more accessible to everyone.

## IDEO-KINETIC FACILITATION AND RELATED BODY-ALIGNMENT TECHNIQUES

These methods originated with the work of Mable Todd and were further developed by Dr. Lulu Sweigard and Barbara Clark. The skeleton is brought into proper alignment for greater ease in movement through the reeducation of the muscles. These techniques teach you to relax and to move in more efficient ways through concentration on movement images. The student often only imagines movement without actually doing it. Later he will do very small movements with intense concentration in order to develop new neuromuscular habits for balanced and efficient initiation and performance of any movement, however complex or particular.

## THE BARTINIEFF FUNDAMENTALS

The Bartinieff Fundamentals of Movement is a method of identifying and improving alignment and movement habits. This approach, developed by Irmgard Bartinieff, draws from her professional experience as a physical therapist and Laban Movement analyst and teacher. The Fundamentals emphasize the importance of the connection and integration of various parts of the body during movement. The Bartinieff Fundamentals method is an integral part of the training program for certification as an Effort/Shape Movement* Analyst. This program is offered only by the Laban Institute of Movement Studies and requires one year of intensive study concluding with a final examination. A graduate of the program becomes a certified Effort/Shape Movement Analyst. A list of those certified in Effort/Shape Analysis who have specialized in teaching the Bartinieff Fundamentals can be obtained by contacting the Laban Institute of Movement Studies, Inc., 151 West 19th Street, New York, N.Y. 10011.

## THE BENJAMIN SYSTEM
## OF MUSCULAR THERAPY

Muscular Therapy is a system of treatment, exercise, and education. It works to reduce excess tension and teach people how to prevent its return. The main objective of Muscular Therapy is to teach people how to keep their own bodies relaxed, aligned, and healthy. It combines several approaches: deep-massage treatments, tension-release impact exercises to aid in the reduction of tension, a series of body-care techniques to help people maintain their new low levels of tension, and its own method of postural-alignment reeducation (outlined in part in Chapter 9 of this book). Practitioners are trained in a three-year program at the Muscular Therapy Institute and are certified by the Muscular Therapy Board of Examiners. For further information, write to Muscular Therapy Institute, Inc., 910 West End Avenue, New York, N.Y. 10025.

*Effort/Shape is a system of analyzing and understanding movement in very specific ways.